How to Operate Your Body

How to Operate Your Body

THE MANUAL LIFE DOESN'T GIVE YOU

William C. Tracy

Space Wizard Science Fantasy
Raleigh, NC
www.spacewizardsciencefantasy.com

Publisher's Note: This publication is designed to provide accurate and authoritative information in regard to the subject matter covered. This book is not intended as a substitute for the medical recommendation of physicians or other healthcare providers. Rather, it is intended to offer information to help the reader cooperate with physicians and health professionals in a mutual quest for optimum well-being. You should consult with your physician or other professional(s) when appropriate. Neither the publisher nor the author shall be liable for any personal injury, loss of profit, or any other commercial damages, including but not limited to special, incidental, consequential, personal, or other damages.

Cover art by MoorBooks
Editing by Heather Tracy
Pictures Copyright © 2023, 2025 by Josiah Brooks, Courtney Brooks, and William C. Tracy
Book Layout © 2015 BookDesignTemplates.com

How to Operate Your Body /William C. Tracy.— 1st ed.
ISBN 978-1-960247-39-1

Author's website: www.spacewizardsciencefantasy.com

Dedicated to all those Sunday practice sessions. I keep learning, and I keep discovering how much I don't know.

CONTENTS

Foreword

This is your meat-bag.
No one gave you a manual.
Let's learn how it works.

There is a simple revelation in the haiku above: life does not, in fact, give you a manual. However, we as humans have conquered many challenges. We've created and recorded vast stores of knowledge. We have redefined ourselves and continue to advance in math, science, engineering, history, art, law, etc.

We will spend months or years learning a new skill. We pride ourselves on learning some piece of newly invented technology. But very few of us spend time learning how our bodies operate. But are our bodies not our own, personal, machines? We learn how to modify our computers and upgrade them. We buy the latest new technology or games to get that new thrill, but when a part of our body underperforms, we just run to a doctor or shrug it off.

Your body is as capable as the newest technology. It's time to make it better, faster, stronger.

I'm William C. Tracy, and I've spent the last twenty years working in the field of body mechanics. I have a master's in mechanical engineering, specializing in linkage dynamics, and have been active in martial arts since 2002. The two fields may not seem related, but together they allowed for a journey of investigation into how my body operates mechanically, energetically, and practically.

Now, some twenty years later, I have many years as a performance engineer at a major construction company behind me. During that time, I worked on kinematic systems (how things move with and against each other), and control systems (keeping complex systems in balance). I've worked nearly as long teaching martial arts.

In the past decade, I received instruction from some really excellent martial artists, including: Hironori Otsuka III, the grandmaster of Wado Ryu Karate (my discipline);

Sensei Matthew Harlan, 5th Dan in Wado Ryu Karate and our direct teacher; David Gimberline, an instructor of Shotokan, Shoto Ryu, Goshin Justsu, and practical karate applications; and Elmar Schmeisser, a karate instructor with over fifty years of experience in multiple martial arts disciplines, as well as neurophysiology.

Along with learning from these instructors, I've focused on the fine methods of control for each musculature system in the body, incorporating them into my teaching style. I certainly haven't learned everything, but I don't intend to stop.

However, in this book, I'm not going to teach you martial arts, how to punch, kick, or how to attack people. Instead, I'm going to teach you how to *move and understand your body.*

Moving—putting one foot in front of the other, picking up something heavy, reaching for an object, or just getting out of the bed in the morning—is not something we often think about. But it's incredibly important. Many causes of sore shoulders and rotator cuffs, bad backs, painful legs, and tight necks lie in poor posture and inefficient movement.

However, that's not the biggest thing this book will teach you. It will teach you how to move *efficiently.* There is a big difference in efficient motion and just moving. The stability and efficiency of the upper half of the body depends on a solid base in the bottom half.

Periodically, I'll ask you to do exercises. If you follow along and try them out, you'll have a much better time understanding what I'm saying. My advice is to do them, even if you think you understand the principles already. One of my favorite moments in martial arts is when a student starts practicing a simple concept I've nagged them about for years, then is surprised it works! Really, try things out and I think you'll be surprised.

To temper that, I have a quick *I Am Not a Doctor* warning. Much of the knowledge presented in this book comes from experimentation and observation over many years, but I don't have a degree or license in physical therapy, or medicine. I'll give you, the reader, the warning I give my karate students: **don't do something if it hurts**. Human bodies are all different, with large ranges of shapes and flexibilities. If an exercise I suggest hurts or seems impossible for you, don't do it! At the very least, approach with caution. Use your own discretion, especially if you have a specific limitation. There are also differences in bodies with more estrogen and ones with more testosterone. These are the hormones that express female and male characteristics, and some of those affect how the body moves! In response to feedback on the original book, I've tried to introduce more models in the pictures (i.e. not just me, a white male), to show differences.

Finally, if these explanations and examples help you, there's no big secret, so please pass these methods on to others who might need them! I've done a lot of trial and error over the years so you don't have to. If I can ease a little pain and help more people live to their full potential, I'll be happy. Alright. Enough of this introduction. Let's learn How to Operate Your Body.

William C. Tracy
January 2025

Correct Posture

Hips, Shoulders, Back, Knees, Feet, and Head

Operating your body well is no easy matter. Imagine that you are an infant. You don't know how to move your arms or your legs, or really how to do anything. Pretend you are discovering your body's limits for the very first time. It's much easier to learn something new rather than relearn, but coming at a new technique with an open mind helps bridge that gap.

One of the core problems, and one of the most easily corrected issues with body mechanics, is posture. Having good posture is essential to learning concepts introduced later in this book, like how to walk efficiently. Seriously, if you keep only one lesson from this book, work on posture.

We often get so used to doing an action a certain way that it feels alien to do it any other way. I may ask you to undo something you're used to or at least try a different method. It's as uncomfortable as eating or brushing your

So, you want to feel better and get in shape, right? Does your back hurt when you play video games, or do your hips ache after a day at the office? This is the book for you! Instead of telling you what weights to lift at the gym, this book will give you some simple exercises to get you feeling better and moving quicker. After you're moving efficiently, then you can decide if you want to hit the gym!

This book is divided into a few sections:

1) Basic definitions, posture, and stretching.
2) Anatomy of the body
3) Cool techniques to learn!

I'd highly recommend going through the anatomy sections before you get to the Cool Things because I'll be referencing what you've learned.

teeth with your non-dominant hand. But give it a try. At least by changing your posture you won't get toothpaste all over your face.

Before we get to how to operate your body correctly, we're going to build up some good habits to make the final sections of this book easier to understand. Stay with me and I promise we'll get there!

For learning posture, let's take this from the head down. The bulbous cabbage sitting on top of your shoulders can weigh as much as a bowling ball. If this bowling ball is sticking out in front of you, rather than being directly above your body, you'll be predisposed to moving where the bowling ball leads you.

First exercise! If you have a bowling ball, use that, but if not, get something else that weighs about 15 pounds (that's about 7 kg for those using the metric system). Hold the object directly in front of you, cradling it with your hands, touching your stomach around your bellybutton. You'll feel the weight, but it probably won't be too much of an imposition. That's because where you're holding it is very close to your center of mass.

Ah. I should step back and explain the center of mass.

If you want to be technical about it, the way to find the center of mass is this: take an object, wrap it with a piece of string from one end to another, then hang it up on a wall. Draw a line along the length of the string. Now, take the same object, wrap the string around a different length, and hang it up again a different way. Draw another line. If you do this several different times, the center of mass will be where all the lines cross. Let's use Vitty the Vitruvian Man as an example. You can see in Figure 1 how the vertical line

> With each new section you go through in this book, you will feel differences in posture, body connections from your feet to your shoulders, and of course, how you walk. Take the time to really understand what's going on, and when each change starts to gel, then it's time to move on to the next section.

describes his center of mass when hung up in different directions.

Granted, you're probably not going to wrap yourself up in string and tape yourself to the wall. If you do, please send me pictures.

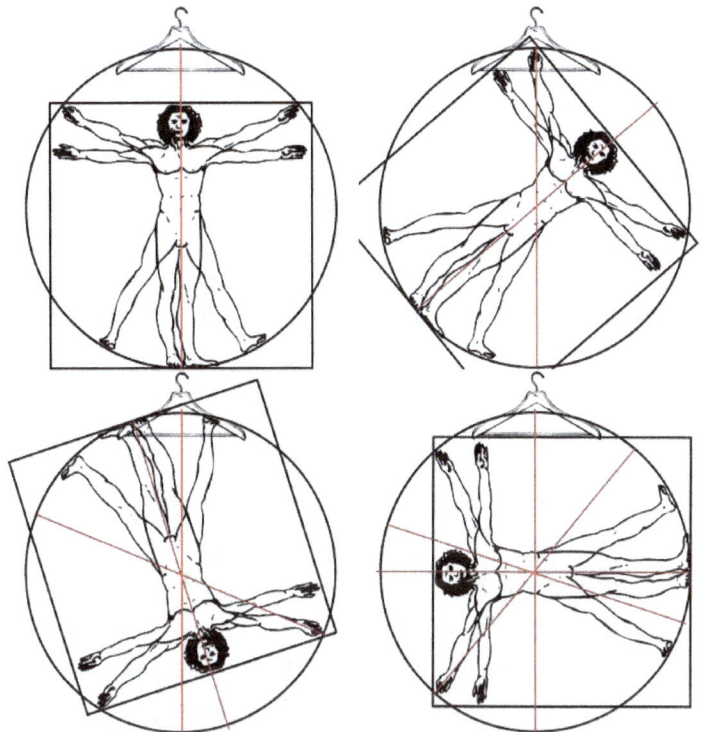

Figure 1: Vitty is hung up by his head, arms, legs, and side to determine his center of mass.

For now, take my word for it that your center of mass—assuming you own two arms, two legs, your head, and you're standing upright—is right around your bellybutton.

So, you're standing there with a bowling ball held at your center of mass. You're still holding the bowling ball, right? No? Well, pick it up again.

As I said, when you hold this at your center of mass, it doesn't affect your balance much because the mass is concentrated where you carry mass all the time. Try reaching your hands forward so your elbows are at your stomach and the bowling ball is out in front of you. It feels a lot heavier, doesn't it? Now, try lifting the ball up so you're holding it at the same height as your head, directly in front of you. You feel like you're going to fall forward, right? Now you can put the ball down.

When you stand upright and your head is not directly above your body, the situation is the same as holding a bowling ball in front of your face. You're predisposed to moving forward, rather than any other direction. But since you're used to doing so, you don't notice your body's bias. To be able to move efficiently, you want to start from a true neutral stance. Let's continue correcting that bias.

Second exercise. Bring your head back so your ears are directly above your shoulders. Make sure you don't raise your chin when you do this (and don't push your shoulders

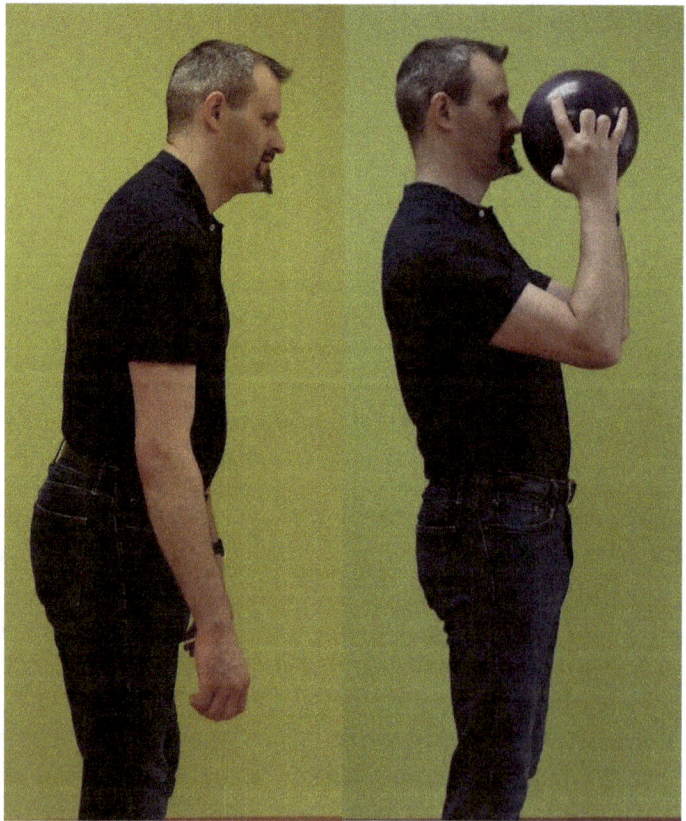

Figure 2: A bowling ball held in front of your head simulates the weight of keeping your head forward.

forward either!). Keep your eyes level so you're not looking down your nose. You may feel a slight pressure in your neck if it's not used to this position. If you're standing up, you may even start to tip backward because you're used to holding your head forward all the time. Not falling over means you're learning to compensate for standing up straight.

If I had to guess, I'd suspect after moving your head into a strange position, your shoulders are now bunched up near your ears. Next step, relax your shoulders.

Keep your ears above your shoulders, or rather above the center of your body. While you do this, bring your shoulders up to your ears, like I just said not to. Then push them all the way back as far as they can go. Last, bring your shoulders straight down. To recap, up into your ears, straight back, straight down. This is where your shoulders should be. It may feel like you're really pushing them backward, but again, that's because you're used to keeping them forward.

> If your shoulders are tight, they may crackle when you move them up, back, and down. That's just the synovial fluid getting released from where it's been pent up. Don't worry about it.

Where's your head?

Has it gone forward again? Are you holding a bowling ball up in the air?

Now we have two pieces to put together. Fix your shoulders as above, then fix your head so your ears are above your shoulders. Your chest will protrude when you do this, no matter your gender. That's because this is correct posture. You already look more confident and authoritative. I've used both correct posture and incorrect posture in groups of people. They take more notice and defer to you when you have correct head and shoulder posture. It's as if we know as a social group that if someone can get this detail right, they may know what they're talking about.

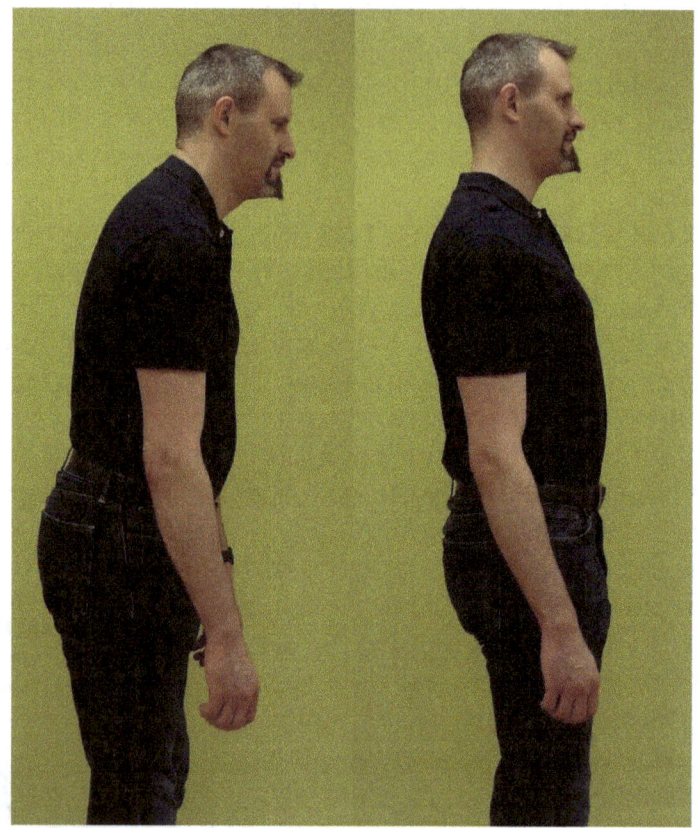

Figure 3: Poor posture (left) vs. correct posture (right). We pay more attention to people with good posture.

Okay, we've fixed the top half, but what about the rest? Positioning your upper body directly over your legs will make it much easier to walk more efficiently.

If your lower back hurts, you might be compressing it with poor posture. This part is going to be a little hard to explain, but I'll do my best.

How often do you pay attention to your hips? The answer is: not enough (yes, I'm aware I'm making an assumption...I'm also aware I'm correct). Remember when I talked about your center of mass? What joint is closest to that area? Your hips. Fixing the way your hips work can improve your posture, fix back problems, improve your gait, and much more.

The biggest problem I see with my introductory martial arts students is that their hips are all wrong. The way most of us naturally stand is with our butts pushed out behind us. This is a "lazy" posture. It's lazy because you're not using your muscles. When you stand this way, you can "lock" your lower back, then you don't have to use your core muscles or your back muscles to help you stand. Sure, it takes less energy muscle-wise, but it also puts more strain on the bones and disks of your spine. It's not a coincidence back problems are one of the most common of the human body. If you're not used to keeping a connection in your core, don't worry. We'll have some exercises for that soon.

Try the "lazy" position out, if you don't naturally stand that way. Stand straight, push your butt out, and let your belly relax. Now stop doing it. Since you've experienced this posture, you can do the opposite.

Instead of pushing your butt out behind you, tuck your hips inward. If you have trouble feeling this, try the following: Put your hands on your hips. Align the edge of your forefinger with the vertical seam of your pants. The more you stick your butt out, the more your finger is going to point behind you. What you want to do is bring your finger forward so it points straight down.

If that doesn't work for you, here's another way to visualize it. Point your forefinger straight out from the button that fastens your pants. Or if you're wearing a belt, straight out from the buckle. Not straight out parallel to the floor, but straight in the direction the button or belt buckle is pointing.

If you're sticking your butt out, then your finger will be pointing slightly down. You want to tuck your hips in until your finger is pointing parallel to the ground. As you do this, you may feel your back lengthen. This is a good sign.

Along with your hips, it's also important to pay attention to your knees. You shouldn't ever lock them out. First, this can hyperextend your knee (that is, extend it more than it should, which will stress your joints), and second, straight knees keep you from adjusting your balance on the fly. Adjusting balance is something we all do naturally. This is partially what makes the Boston dynamics robots' movement seem so natural (or scary). We see a robot kicked, stumble, and right its balance, just as we can. They've managed to program a robot to bend its knees. This will be our downfall.

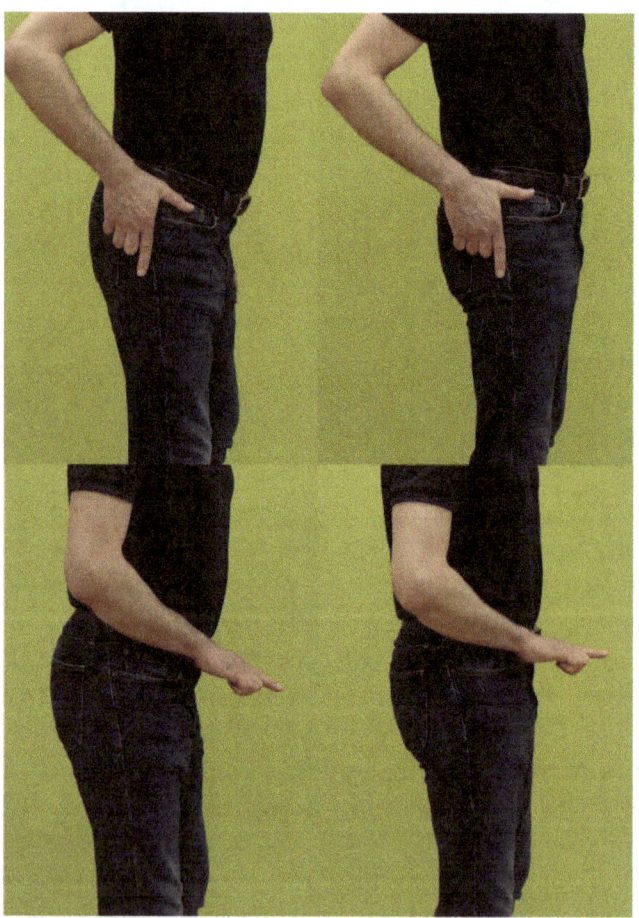

Figure 4: Visualizing alignment in poor posture (left) vs. correct posture (right).

But you too can bend your knees and fight the robot menace! Flexing your knees just a little engages your thigh muscles and lets you react faster to anything that would push you off balance. If you add this to the other three tips above, you will not only have better posture, but be able to hold it better and for longer.

If you do have lower back problems, there's another exercise to help you lengthen your back and stretch it out.

With your good balance (head, shoulders, hips, knees), turn your feet slightly inward (no more than about ten degrees), and let your knees and your hips follow them. Keep your knees above your toes. This opens up your lower back area. While tucking your hips as well as turning your legs toward each other, your back will stretch in two directions. You can add a third stretch if you think about extending outward rather than compressing inward. Pretend your head is tied to the ceiling by a piece of string, keeping your body taut. Reach upward with your head (in good posture, yes).

> Let's put the three exercises together. Are you holding a bowling ball (or object of similar weight) too far forward? First, bring your head back so your ears are above your center of mass. Tuck your chin. Second, get those shoulders out of your ears. Up, back, and down. Third, tuck your hips in so your belt buckle is pointing straight forward. You're well on the way to good posture.

Now, it's time to practice. Set a timer for thirty seconds or set a "good posture reminder" on your phone, if needed. I'm not joking when I suggest every thirty seconds. Or even less. It's at once satisfying and frustrating to feel how much you can straighten up. When your shoulders and neck and hips open up, everything will feel much better. But you'll naturally sag back to a "lazy" posture after a few moments.

You'll feel it every single time your timer goes off, but over time your posture will improve.

I promise it will get easier. The more often you remind yourself to have good posture, and follow through with the exercise above, the more often your body will naturally line up in that position. Over time, you'll be able to increase the reminder time to a minute, two minutes, five ten, half an hour, and more. Eventually, you'll wonder how you ever stood up before.

We'll leave basic posture for now, but I'll be referencing it throughout this book. For now, just keep these four points in mind: *head, shoulders, hips, knees.* You can adjust these while standing or sitting. Try both! If I reference one of these four or tell you to get back to good posture, you'll understand what I mean. You just thought about it again, didn't you? Go ahead and fix your posture one more time before the next section!

> Up to now, I've shown you what to do, but here's the really hard part: unless you actually practice correct posture, you won't do it.

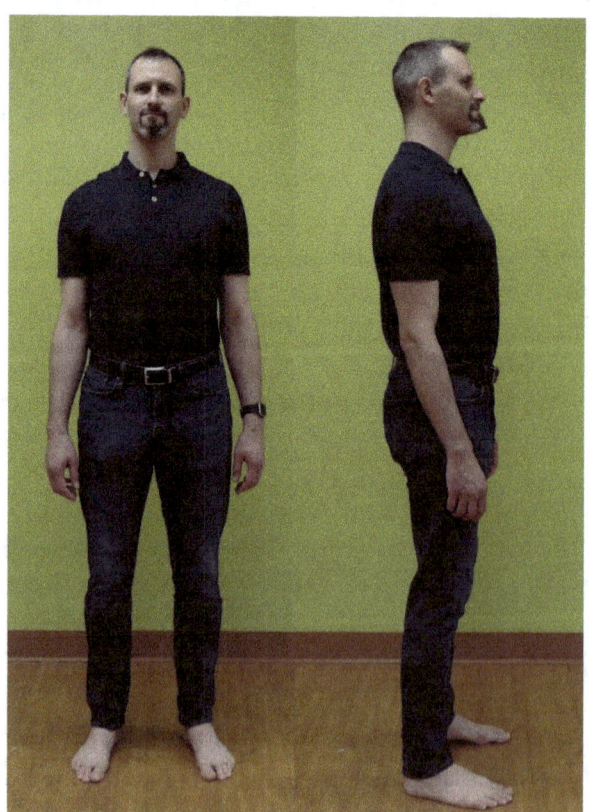

Figure 5: Correct posture, front and side view. Note the head is extended upward, as if connected to the ceiling with string.

Learning About Your Center

I talked briefly about your center above, but I want to go more in depth. Whether you call this your center, your bellybutton, your center of mass, the center of your chi, your tanden or hara, your Dantian, your sacral or svadhishthna chakra, etcetera—people have recognized the significance of this area for thousands of years. It makes sense that it has some importance tied to it. I'm going to leave aside all the metaphysical implications as that could fill another book, and I'm not the correct person to write it.

Instead, I'm going to talk about the physical and mechanical aspects of your center. I say your bellybutton, or refer to your hips moving, but the actual position is about three fingers down from your bellybutton and two fingers inside your body. This is that spot you would find if you hung yourself up a wall with string like Vitty in the last section.

Now you know how to find your center of mass, but why would you want to? Have you ever balanced a pen or spoon or fork on one finger before? You can do this because you are finding its center of mass. The unique property of the center of mass of an object is that if you manipulate the center, you will manipulate the entire object at one time. This is assuming the object you are manipulating is rigid, or at least, does not flex too much. Obviously, your body flexes a lot, as you can move your arms and legs and head in all directions. For right now, I'm talking about your center when your feet are both planted on the floor, about as wide apart as your hips, you have good posture as outlined above (remember your posture!), and your hands are hanging by your sides.

How do you get to know your center? First, you need to have good posture. I know I keep harping on this, but it really is important. Changing your posture will change where your center of mass is. You want your physical center of mass to line up with your metaphysical one (three fingers down and two fingers in from your bellybutton). Feet at hip width, knees slightly bent, hips tucked, shoulders back and down, ears in line with your shoulders. Extend your body as if your head is hanging by a string from the ceiling.

> If you get really good at finding the center of objects, you can do astounding feats like balancing circular objects on top of one another, or juggling six or seven balls, or doing several complicated actions at once. That takes a lot of practice, although it is fun to do.

Whew! That's a lot. But keep at it. Getting into that position will become second nature, especially if you keep doing it every time I mention it while you read this book. Do you have a timer running?

In good posture, your center is aligned. Now let's play with it. We are going to move different body parts around to show you how much effect it has on your center. First, from good position, put both arms out in front of you, relaxed, at the height of your shoulders, as if you've become a zombie and want a brain sandwich. Then push both shoulders forward and reach out as far as you can with your hands. Get those brains! As you do this, you'll start toppling forward. Reset and try it again. Feel free to stagger and moan and see if anyone hits you with a baseball bat.

The arms are the easiest to try this exercise with because they make the largest change in your center of mass from a standing position. Let's try two others and see if you can feel the difference. Get back in a good posture (remember to tuck those hips!), and start leaning your head forward, as if you are a turtle poking out of your shell. This simulates holding that bowling ball in front of your face. You may have to go farther than you would using your arms before you start falling forward, because your head doesn't reach as far (I hope!).

One more. Get back in a good position, especially making sure to tuck your hips under you, because this is what we're going to move. Start pointing your pants button or belt buckle downward and stick your butt out, and feel when you begin falling backward. If you've got a "lazy" posture, this is the difference you have to contend with while walking around. It's quite significant.

The reason these small motions make such a difference is because you are aligned with your center of mass and, like balancing a pencil on your finger, you have very fine control over your body. These are simple examples, and you can play on your own by adjusting both your posture, and where your arms and legs are.

> You'll find your balance gets a lot better when your center is aligned. For example, standing on one foot is a lot easier with good posture.

I'll get to more applications of controlled movement closer to end of the book, but for now, pay attention to a few things while you move around, at least until you're comfortable with good posture. The first is that when you are aligned over your center, in good posture, you will be lighter on your feet. This happens because you don't have to account for being off balance while your head is forward or your hips are misaligned. Second, try things like walking up hills while you have good posture. I bet it will be easier! I'll leave you to play with this for now, but I'll come back to it again later. For now, don't lose your posture! Head, shoulders, hips, knees.

In fact, if you've read up to here from the beginning, this is a good place to take a break before we get to more complicated actions. Practice standing with your timer. See if you can get up to 30 seconds without losing your posture. Do you have good posture both while standing and sitting? Are your shoulders relaxed? Remember what I said at the beginning of this chapter? If you only take one thing away from this book, take this one: good posture will fix a lot of things by itself.

Moving Around

Muscles, Ligaments and Tendons

Now you understand a bit about how your body is affected by your posture and center of mass, I want to talk about the way your body is internally connected. You've probably heard this in high school biology, so I'm not going to go too in-depth.

First, muscles. Basically, muscles are a soft tissue made of protein, where strands slide past each other so the muscle can contract and release. These are the things that connect your bones together and enable you to stand up. Without them, you wouldn't be able to move and would collapse in a pile.

This section will have a lot of exercises that are good to practice on a regular basis. They will help keep your body flexible and strong. Being proficient at them will also better enable you to try out the more complex actions at the end of the book.

There are several different types of muscle, including cardiac muscle in your heart, the smooth muscle in your internal organs, and skeletal muscle—that is the muscle that binds your skeleton together. The first two muscle types are largely involuntary. That is, you have no control over them. Instead, let's talk about where you *do* have control. Having control means you can improve in those areas, especially if you haven't tried before.

Learning how your muscles move is the basis for understanding how to operate your body. Play around with how your body moves. Open and close your hands. See how it affects your forearm. Move your foot up and down, and see how it affects your lower leg and calf. Sit and stand while you put your hands on your butt, to see how your gluteus muscles contract and expand. Basically, go touch yourself a lot (not a euphemism). You'll learn some things.

Two other types of tissue that are intertwined (literally) with muscles are ligaments and tendons. People often confuse these, if they even know what they are. If you've ever seen an anatomy diagram, you usually see a muscle colored in red. You also may see another bit of something colored in white that attaches to or emerges from the muscle. This is usually the connective tendon.

Tendons are tough bands of tissue, sort of like rubber bands, and while they don't contract and expand as much as muscle fibers do, they are the things that let your muscles work with your skeleton. A tendon emerges from a muscle and connects to one of the nearby bones, acting as an anchor. Imagine you have a bunch of bones, and you want to figure out how to make them move around. You could blow up a balloon halfway so that the shape is malleable—long and thin or short and round. This is sort of how a muscle moves. But then how do you connect that balloon to your bones? Cut a rubber band, tie one end around the neck of the balloon, and tie the other end around one of the bones. Tape the top of the balloon to another bone. The rubber band lets the balloon flex. You have the equivalent of a tendon. Tendons are tough, can resist a lot of stress, but can tear if they are moved in the wrong direction or stretched too far. The Achilles tendon is one of the easiest ones to find in your body. Sit down and bring one foot up in front of you or rest it on your other leg. Put your thumb on the area between your heel and your ankle, then move your foot up and down. You'll feel a thick band there that tenses and relaxes as you move your foot. If you move your fingers up your leg, you can feel how the Achilles tendon interacts with your muscle all the way up to your calf, right below your knee. So, tendons are like thick rubber bands attaching muscle to bone.

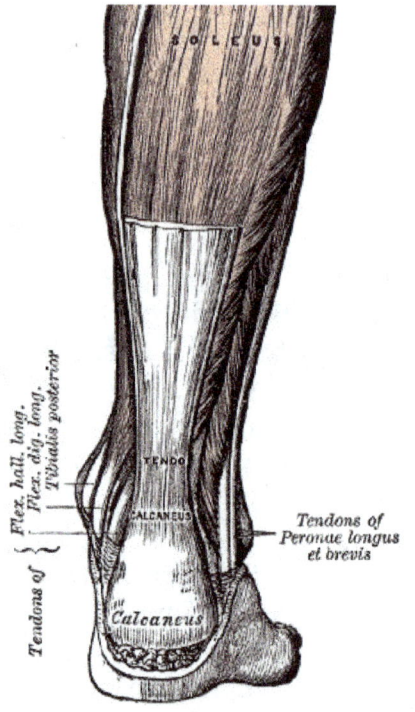

Figure 6: The Achilles Tendon (*Gray's Anatomy*).

Ligaments, on the other hand (or *in* the other hand, right? Right?), are much more static than tendons, because ligaments connect bones to other bones. There is little expansion and contraction like there is in a muscle. Just like a tendon, a ligament can be torn from an injury, from overexertion, or from moving your body in a way that it's not supposed to move. If you want to feel a ligament, again sit down, but this time put both feet on the floor. Put a hand on one knee and let your fingers rest right beneath your kneecap. You will feel a thick band of tissue. If you swing your lower leg up then back to the floor, you can feel this band of tissue as it flexes a small amount between your leg bone and your kneecap. It doesn't move nearly as much as your Achilles tendon does. Ligaments don't move as much as tendons because bones generally stay in the same place in our bodies, unlike muscles. However, ligaments also take longer to heal because your bones grow a lot slower than your muscles do. What you're feeling under your kneecap is the patellar ligament (often called the patellar tendon, but that's technically wrong, and now you know why!)

Behind that, *inside* your knee is yet another ligament. If you've heard of someone with a torn ACL, that's the anterior cruciate *ligament,* and it will often never repair on its own, instead needing surgery. Don't mess around with your ligaments. You need them!

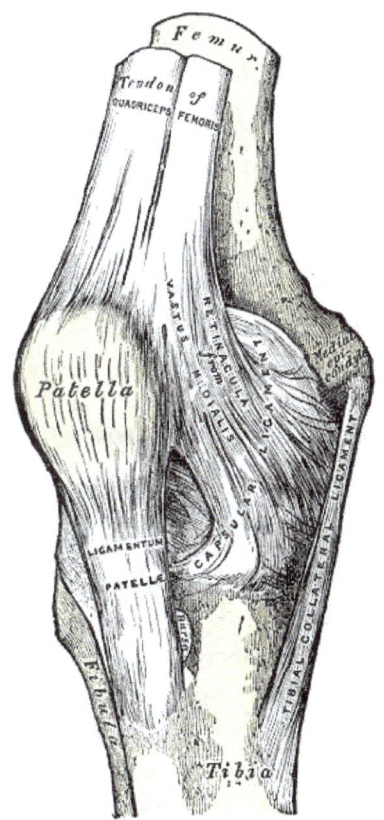

Figure 7: The patellar ligament (*Gray's Anatomy*). The ACL is inside the knee joint, connecting the femur and tibia.

Again, I encourage you to feel your own body. Where a part of you bends (arms, legs, waist, neck, etc.), put a hand on the area that moves the most as you bend. You can feel

> Changing the way your body moves, especially if you're adopting a new way of standing (with correct posture), can lead to more stress on muscles that aren't used to the load. You might find your shoulders or back hurt *more* the first few days of using correct posture. As always, make certain what you are doing is correct posture, and you're not introducing a new imbalance or compensation. It's ok to take breaks from this new posture but try to add a little more time each day. Soon you'll get used to it, and I promise good posture will lead to fewer aches and pains in the long run. A good way to make that happen sooner is in the next section.

all these little connections. A great example is your shoulder, because it moves in all directions. Put a hand on your opposite shoulder and move your arm around. You'll feel a bunch of muscles, tendons, and ligaments all moving in your shoulder joint. Discovering what's happening is one of the best ways to learn how to operate your body.

Pain and Discomfort

There are a few things to go over before we get to stretching, anatomy, and the cool things I can show you about your body. The first is pain. What is it? We've all experienced it. At some point, you've said, "Ow, that hurts." Pain comes from a few different places and causes, but we all experience it a little differently. A lot of the time we can see a direct cause, especially with acute, sharp pain. Suffering an injury causes what's called *nociceptive* pain, from obvious tissue or bone damage. There is also *neuropathic* pain, caused by nerve damage resulting from disease or degeneration, and *nociplastic* pain, which is linked to changes in the way the body processes pain. We don't actually understand why we feel some types of pain, and why some people feel it more intensely than others. Sometimes pain can actually result from social or emotional factors. I'm not going to go in-depth with this, save to say that it's a valuable part of how to operate your body. Pain tells you something is wrong. Let's just say you generally want to avoid pain, because even if there's nothing obvious, it might be the precursor of something much worse.

In contrast, we also feel soreness or discomfort. What's the difference? Pain is also discomfort, right? Well, yes and no. Soreness is not usually acute or sharp like the pain we feel from cuts or breaks, and it doesn't last for weeks or months like chronic pain or the pain from nerve regrowth, though it might last a few days. We often feel soreness or discomfort from doing things a different way than we're used to (like correcting bad posture) or from muscle fatigue (after exercise). Muscles grow by gaining micro-tears during exercise, and these will cause soreness until the muscle recuperates. If you use muscles you have never used much, expect some soreness, but that's ok! If it persists past a few days, then maybe have someone check it out. The remedy might be as simple as stretching or a backrub.

> Remember: Soreness and pain are different, but one can lead to the other. Be aware of your body however you move, in old ways or new ones.

Why is all this important for how to operate your body? Because it's important to know whether the new exercise you're practicing is causing *discomfort* or *pain.* You'll come across new ways of thinking about movement below, so keep these definitions in mind. When there is a different, uncomfortable, feeling in your body, question it. Is it soreness from a new way of moving, or pain from damage? Be aware as well how soreness can cause pain! For example, if you use better posture, you'll be putting a different type of strain on your shoulders, making them sore in new ways for a time. This can, in turn, cause you to move your neck awkwardly and might cause stiffness or actual pain! Keep all this in the back of your mind while you learn the cool things I have to show you and make sure not to overreach!

The Importance of Small Muscles

The little muscles, or support muscles, are vitally important to having a well-balanced body. Many fitness books, weightlifting programs, and even some personal trainers skip over this, but it's dangerous to do so. These small sections of larger muscles help out as you move, providing stabilization and control. If you are trying to increase your muscle mass (which is by no means required to get a lot out of this book), a lot of training programs will focus on making the big muscles bigger, because they're more impressive aesthetically. However, big muscles without a good support staff can lead to joint problems in the future. It's like trying to run a large business with only a CEO. You need employees to support and carry out the decisions made by the person at the top.

Instead of being able to lift a large weight in one direction, I've found it's more useful to lift a normal or light weight in *any* direction with full control. Jugglers don't juggle extremely heavy objects, except for quick stunts with bowling balls and chainsaws. Usually, they juggle light balls or pins. They develop full control over them. If you watch an accomplished juggler walk around or do tricks while still juggling several balls, and wonder how they do that, *this* is how. They have small muscular control. Be like the juggler. In fact, we'll cover a bit of how jugglers move toward the end of the book.

Unless you are already used to lifting heavy weights—which most people aren't—you might find a different type of exercise more helpful. Performing slow, controlled exercises can be very beneficial.

Once you have developed small muscles, then work on making the big muscles bigger if you wish. With large muscles buoyed by a support staff of small muscles, you have a much-reduced chance of joint injury. As I've detailed above, you *really* don't want to have an injured joint. Tendons take a long time to heal. Ligaments may never heal without surgery. They are one of the worst injuries to have, especially for someone in an active sport. While bones heal and can even become denser with trauma, ligaments and tendons take an agonizingly long time to heal—on the order of months or even years.

Here are a couple simple exercises to show you—even if you are used to lifting a lot of weight—how useful it is to develop small muscle mass.

Wall push-ups: stand a couple feet out from a wall, facing it. Raise your arms so you can comfortably place your palms on the wall, while allowing just a little bit of flex in your elbows. Remember your good posture from the first chapter! Get your shoulders back, your head back, and tuck your hips in. Now, while keeping all those parts aligned, slowly bend your elbows to bring your face closer to the wall, making sure your arms stay as close to your sides as possible. That is, don't let them pop out like chicken wings. Bend only your elbows, keeping everything else in place, so that when you finish, your bent elbows will be right above the tops of your hips, as in Figure 8. Go slow! Keep your good alignment as you do the push-up. Be certain not to let your hips untuck, because this means you're going to put extra pressure on your lower back. If you need a reminder, look at Figure 4 again. Untucked hips also mean you are no longer connected between your hips and your shoulders, which means you're not exercising the muscles you should. To get the full motion, try to bend your arms until the tip of your nose touches the wall. Then come back up to your starting position. It's a small, controlled

> Why do push-ups? Because they teach you to have a connected core, which is vital to developing proper coordination between the lower and upper halves of your body.

motion. Resist the urge to go too fast or fling yourself away from the wall. Remember, you're working on small support muscles.

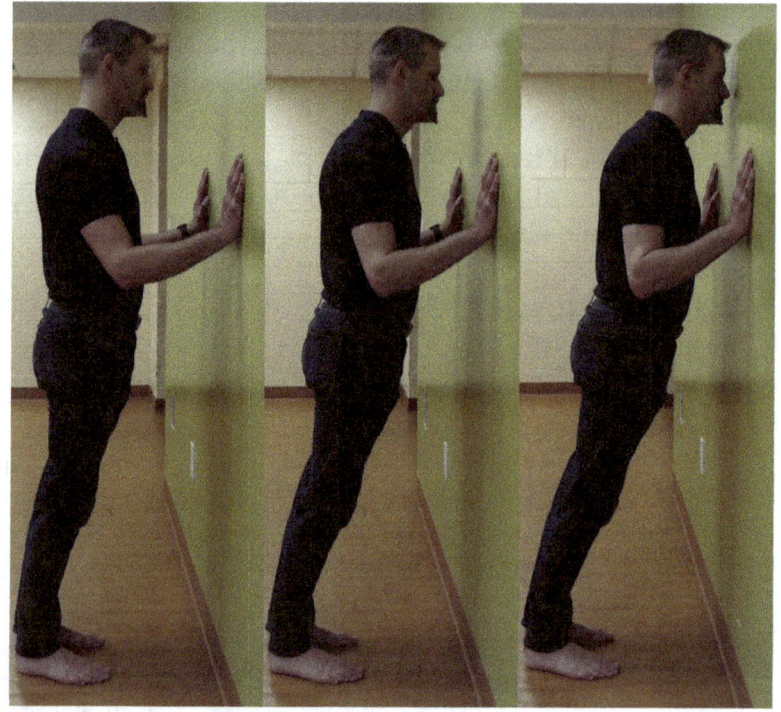

Figure 8: The range of a wall push-up.

Go try this now. Take this book with you and find a wall. Is your posture good? If not, feel free to imagine me shaking a stern finger at you.

...

Did you try it out? You'll get more out of this book if you experience what I'm saying.

Alright. I'm going to assume you did some wall push-ups, but I'm watching you.

Even if you have little to no arm strength, you should be able to do a few wall push-ups. On the other hand, if you are used to doing lots of push-ups or lifting weights, I'd still ask you to try this out and see what you feel. Go extremely slowly, holding a good posture all the way down. Hold for a count of one-one thousand at the wall. Then push yourself up to your starting position at the same (slow) speed. When you do a correct wall push-up, with good posture, you should start to feel some strain and little movements inside your shoulders around the joint.

These little movements mean you are not only using the large muscles of your arm, but also the little muscles around the joints of your elbows and your shoulders. Try to do ten of these wall push-ups three times a week, and you will quickly feel an improvement in the way your joints move. If that works, gradually increase the number you can do by three or four per session. Performing a lot of low-stress exercises will tire you out and thus improve your small muscles.

Try writing a reminder on a Post-it® and sticking it in an annoying place so you remember to practice.

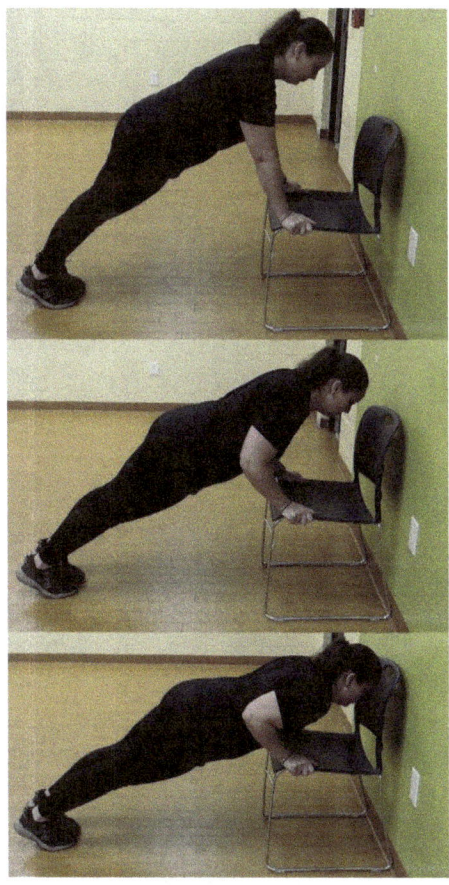

Figure 9: The range of a chair pushup.

If you find wall push-ups too easy or, better yet, if you've been trying them out for a week or two, you might try chair push-ups instead. These are basically the same thing, except you're leaning at a deeper angle than a wall push-up to start. First find a sturdy chair, the higher the better. Don't use a swivel chair because that's just going to throw you off to one side and I'll laugh. Now, grasp the sides of the chair seat with your arms extended and your feet on the floor. Using good posture, slowly lower yourself down until you're right above the chair seat. Push back up. Repeat.

Wall squats: while wall push-ups work on your elbows and your shoulders, this less intensive version of a squat will help you learn the small muscles around your hips and knees. In the upper body version of this, your shoulders are the ones benefiting most from improving the smaller muscles. In the lower body version, your knees will see the most benefit.

For this one, stand a little farther than one of your own foot's length away from a wall. You can check by placing one foot behind another to make sure you're out far enough. Lean back until your butt touches the wall. Again, using good posture—hips tucked, shoulders back, head back—slowly slide down the wall as far as you are able. If you are not used to squats, this may be only a few inches. If you are, it might be to where your thighs are horizontal to the floor, or even lower.

> If you have not done squats a lot, I would advise only going down a few inches, certainly no further than where your thighs are horizontal.

The first time you try this, feel where your weight is in your feet. If it's mostly in your toes, then slide your feet out some. You want all the weight in your heels. You should *not* do squats where your weight is in your toes. That can cause injuries to your knee joints.

Once you are used to this exercise you can experiment with going down a few inches farther each time, until your butt is almost touching the floor. Remember to increment your squat *slowly*!

Alright, same drill. Take this book and go test it out. See what you feel. I'll wait here until you're done.

No cheating!

...

If you do this in the correct posture, you should feel more stress on your knees and right above your knees than on your hips, simply because your hips are more used to bending while you walk. Did you feel all the little muscles activating around your knees? This is what you want to develop. With stronger support muscles surrounding your knee, you can resist your knee going the wrong direction or bending farther than it should if you step badly. Squats also help your knees support more weight. Try to do ten of these three times a week and see what improvement you feel.

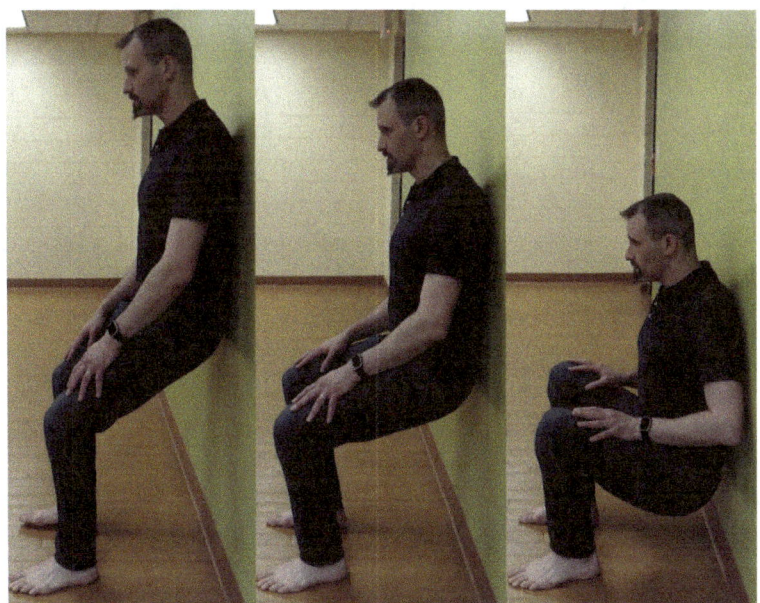

Figure 10: The range of a wall squat. Going past horizontal is the more advanced version.

For both of these exercises, if you find them to be beneficial, slowly increase the number of repetitions over time until you get to twenty. For the push-ups, you can also step your feet further from the wall over time. For the squats, go a few inches deeper toward the floor over time. If you continue to do these exercises, you will strengthen your small muscles. They will then be able to help you out both in day-to-day motion and in strenuous exercising or bodybuilding.

> Add wall squats to that annoying note you have pasted to your phone, your computer monitor, or your forehead.

Stretching

There is some debate on what you do when you stretch, whether you are increasing the flexibility of a tendon, or just the muscle, or some combination of the two. I'm not going to worry about that much here. Suffice to say if you stretch, you will increase your range of motion. However, it is also possible to overstretch and damage something. It's as important to stretch the correct way as it is to stretch at all.

> At the end of this chapter, I'll give you the stretching sequence I teach to office-dwellers to keep them from hunching up like little toads at their computers.

Stretching out your muscles allows you to operate your body to its full extent of motion. I usually do some amount of stretching every day, but if you'd rather have a more focused stretching session three or four times a week, that should be sufficient. You'll notice increased blood flow, better energy, and better flexibility by stretching regularly.

We'll be focusing on the whole body through this section, from the head to the toes. Otherwise, the part not stretched will feel cramped up compared to the rest of your body. I know. I'm making you move around. It's awful. This is one of those things where you'll feel better after you do it.

How do you stretch? There are a few different ways. One is simple static stretching. This is where you hold the position close to the extent of your range of motion for several seconds. Whichever muscle you are stretching may feel looser afterward and move a little easier. There is also dynamic stretching, where you move more quickly through the maximum and minimum range of motion of a joint, but don't hold the extents. Finally, there are a couple niche warm-ups and stretches called isometrics and pandiculation. Read on to learn about these fancy words!

Static stretching

Static stretching is the most common form of stretching and the easiest one to learn. Any place your joint naturally moves, you can go to the extent of that motion to stretch the muscle that connects to the joint. Some of the ones I like are shown below. Try them out one at a time while you go through the description. Some you can do while seated. Others you will have to stand for.

People often carry a lot of stress in their neck and shoulders. These stretches can help release that stress or keep it from getting worse. We'll go over some other techniques to help muscle pain in the section on neck anatomy.

Neck stretch: standing in good posture (head, shoulders, hips, and knees—yes, I know I'm repeating myself. Are you still slumping?), turn your neck to the left to its full range of motion. Hold for a count of one-one thousand. For an added stretch, still in good posture, you can rotate your left shoulder behind you, also rotating your torso, which will give an added stretch. Hold your hips as straight as possible when doing this. Then come back to a neutral position and do the same stretch to the right. Next, from that neutral position, lift your chin until it is pointing as far up as it can without stress. Hold for one count. Then *relax* your neck downward, but be careful not to press your chin into your chest. Pressing down on your neck can cause damage. Last, you can stretch your neck side to side. Hold out your right hand and tilt your head to the left. This will lengthen the tendons in the right side of your neck. If you lower your shoulder and pretend you are reaching for something you can't quite grasp, you will feel a nice stretch in the tendons and muscles that keep your head upright. Repeat with your left hand out and your neck tilted to the right.

Shoulder stretches: Here are some good (but tough) flexibility exercises to increase the range of motion of your shoulders. Since these will potentially be increasing the range of your motion, be careful not to go too fast, and **stop if something hurts**. Understand the difference between stretching and pain, and if you can't move as much as someone else, that's alright. We don't all have the same flexibility.

Let's work on full shoulder rotation. Take your dominant hand first, and reach over your head so your fingers are touching as far below the base of your neck as you can get. Try to reach to your spine in the center of your body. Now move your other hand behind to your lower back and start to creep upward. Can you touch your fingers? Can you lock your fingers? If you can, you can pull a little (not too much) with both arms and stretch your shoulders. Now try the other side. You might have a surprising difference in flexibility between your arms! My left arm can reach higher up my back than my right arm, for example. If you can't touch your hands at all, no problem! Find a short strap, or rope (a belt works great in a pinch) and dangle it down your back with the upper hand. Now you can easily grasp it with the other hand and work your way up as far as is comfortable.

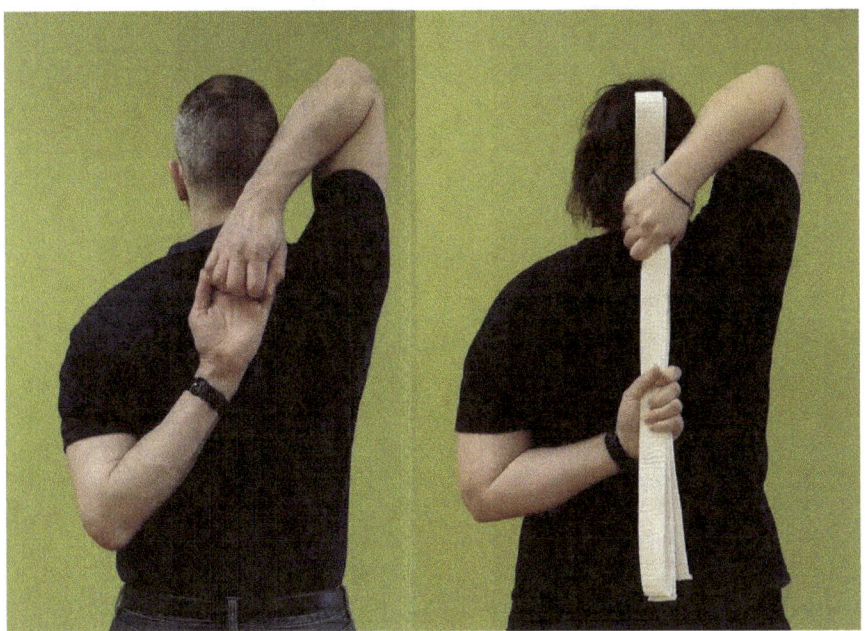

Figure 11: The shoulder stretch exercise with no strap and with a strap.

If you've got that stretch working and need even more, here's a harder one. I have to try this one a couple times myself before I get a good connection, and I'm fairly flexible. This time, put both your hands behind your back, touch your fingertips, then slowly push your hands into each other, aligning along your pinkies, palms, and—if you're flexible enough—all the way so your thumbs are touching and your hands are fully facing and touching behind your back. This is a fantastic stretch to just hold for a few seconds once you get into it. Keeping your shoulders back will help. You should feel this in the front to top of your shoulders, and down into your shoulder blades.

If you can't reach at all, or have trouble getting the flat of your hands touching, try using a strap here as well and holding on to each side behind your back, slowly inching your hands together. If you can touch your hands but can't move them up, try making a fist with both hands instead and touching your knuckles. Then turn your palms down to give more stretch. Pushing your shoulders back (and in good posture) will give a better stretch. Since these are harder stretches, remember always to go slow, and stop if there's any discomfort rather than just a stretching feeling.

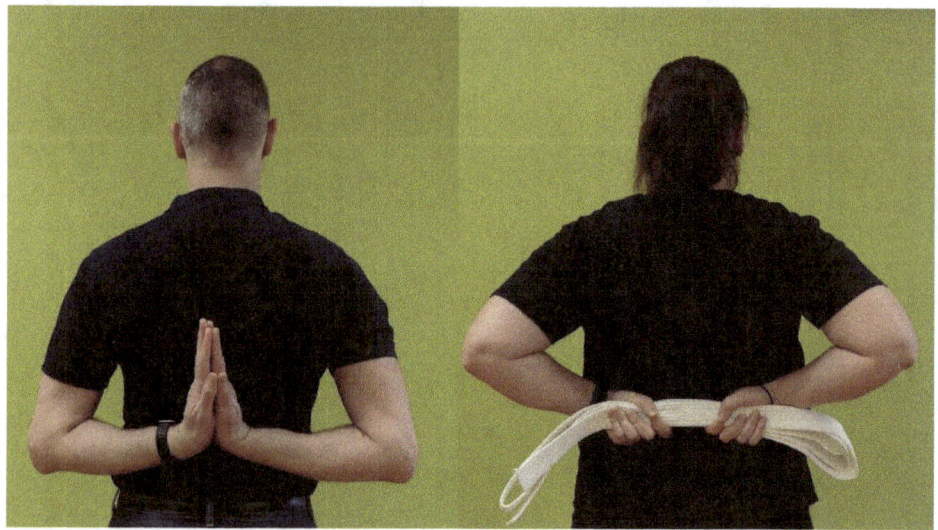

Figure 12: Reverse Prayer with no strap and with a strap.

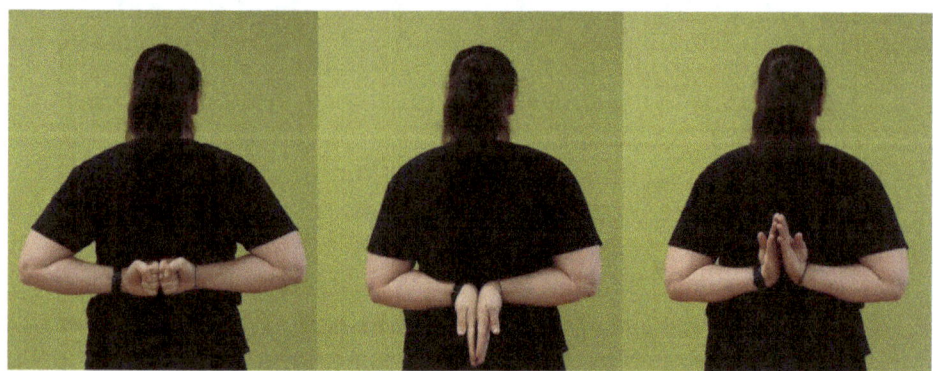

Figure 13: Some alternates for reverse prayer

Arm stretches: put both hands out in front of you, with one hand over top of the other. Extend as far as you can forward, then raise your arms as far as they go while your hands still touch. Then lower them as far as they go while your hands touch. Try to keep your shoulders relaxed as you do this. You can do the same exercise with your arms behind you, although this is more difficult. If you can clasp your hands together behind you, then do so and lift upward until you feel a stretch through your shoulder blades.

If you cannot clasp your hands behind you, then stand next to a wall with one arm behind you and twist your body so your arm stretches in the same manner. Repeat on the other side.

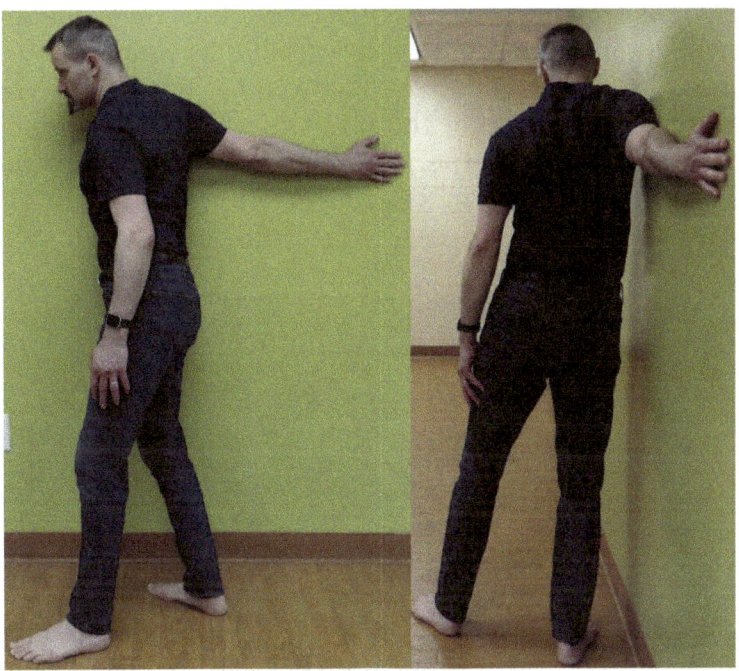

Figure 14: Arm and shoulder blade wall stretch.

Hand stretches: For those of us who primarily work on computers, you're using those fingertips quite a bit! But while you're typing a hundred words a minute, or mousing around in a shooter or action game, or texting with your thumbs, your wrists are actually what are taking the brunt of the stress and pressure. It's why we have a lot of squishy mats for keyboards and fancy mouse rests that help keep us from getting carpal tunnel syndrome. Here are some things you can do to limber up your wrists.

Shake them out! This is one of the easiest ways to get rid of pressure on your wrists. Just remove them from the implement you're manipulating for a few moments and shake out your fingers like there are no towels in the bathroom and you just washed your hands.

Another good wrist stretch is to put a hand straight out in front of you, palm up, then grasp those fingers with the ones of your other hand and pull your hand back toward your elbow. You should feel this all the way up your forearm, and it will open up your carpal tunnel area.

A good general hand stretch is to touch all your fingertips to the ones on the other hand, then press your hands toward each other, stretching out the distance between thumb and index finger while you do. This activates all the little nerves and fascia in your hand.

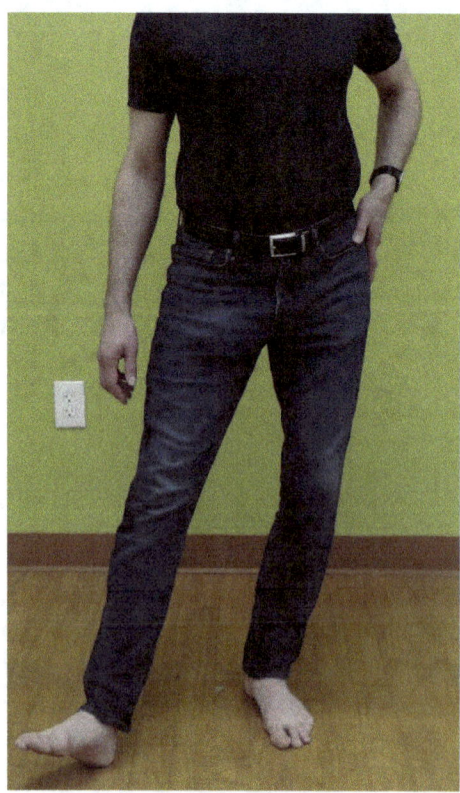

Figure 15: Hip stretch. You can also place your hand on your leg above the knee. You'll feel the stretch where the back hand is shown on the hip.

Hip stretch: this one is easy. Simply stand in good posture, then lean your hip out to one side while keeping your head above your center. You should feel this stretch right below your hipbone on the side you're leaning toward. Hold for a few seconds then repeat on the other side. You can also get a good stretch to the back of your calf if you put the leg opposite to the hip you are stretching out by about a foot, rest on the heel, and lean back. If you need to, lean forward and put one hand above the knee of the leg extended for stability.

Leg stretches, part one: stand in good posture with your feet at hip width, then use your left leg to take a large step out to your left, with your left toes pointing 90 degrees out from your right toes (which you haven't moved). Turn your hips to the left so they are facing the direction you stepped out and bend your left leg. Try to lower your hips into the stretch, which you should feel mainly in your right leg. While you do this, make sure your left knee doesn't go beyond your left toes, as this will cause excess strain in your knee joint. If you look down, you should still be able to see your toes. Repeat on the other side. Try this same thing on both sides again, but after

> Bend your knees and fight the robot menace! Flexing your support knee can give you a lot more balance.

stepping out and turning your hips, also turn your back foot so it is facing the same direction as the front foot. Both feet will be 90 degrees from your original position. Try to press your back heel toward the floor, even if it does not touch, though make sure not to force it or hyperextend. Don't let your knee go past your front toes. This should give a good stretch along the back of your leg. If you need a bigger stretch, step out farther when you start, or sink your hips closer to the ground. Repeat on the other side.

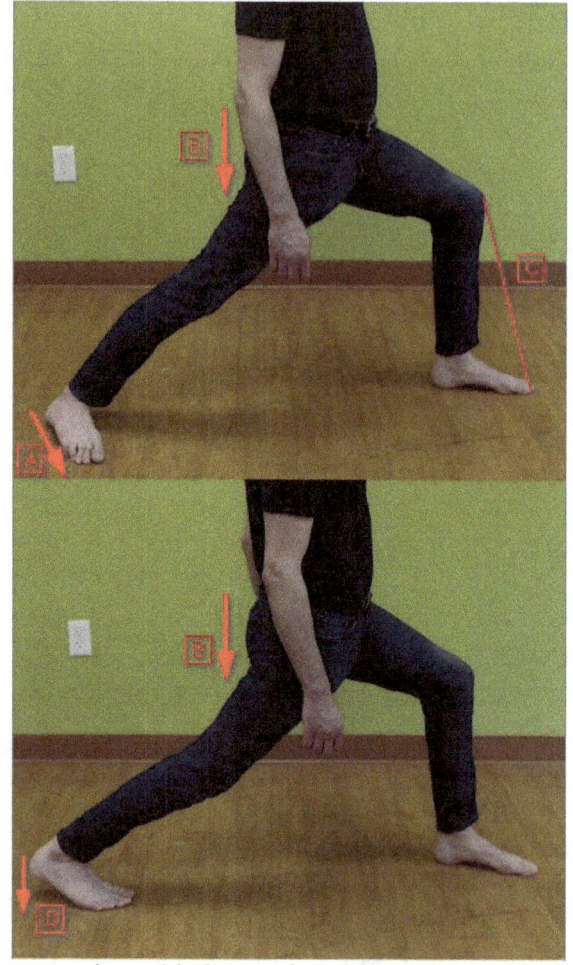

Figure 16: Leg stretches, with the rear foot pointed at 90 degrees (top picture, A) and straight (bottom picture). Sink your hips down in both stretches (B). Don't let your knee go over your foot (C). On the forward stretch, try to sink your rear heel down to the floor (D).

Leg stretches, part two: hold the wall, or a table, or the back of a chair if you need to for stability. This one requires a bit more balance. On the other hand, if you want more challenge, don't hold onto anything, and make this a balance exercise too. Just don't fall over!

While standing on one leg, pull the other knee up straight, as close as you can to your chest, holding with one hand. Count for about eight to ten seconds, then push your knee across your body for another eight to ten seconds, then to the outside for another eight to ten seconds. Next, let your knee drop until it points downward, and grasp your ankle with your hand. Pull your ankle up behind you. You should feel this stretch your quadriceps. If that doesn't work, try pushing your hips forward while you do this. Lastly (and this one takes even more balance and muscle, so don't worry if you can't hold it for long), hold your leg out straight in front of you and try to grab your toes with your hand. Make sure to bend your other knee while you do this for balance. Work on increasing the time you can hold each position until you get to twelve to fifteen seconds.

Whew! That was a lot of work! Only one more static stretch to go...

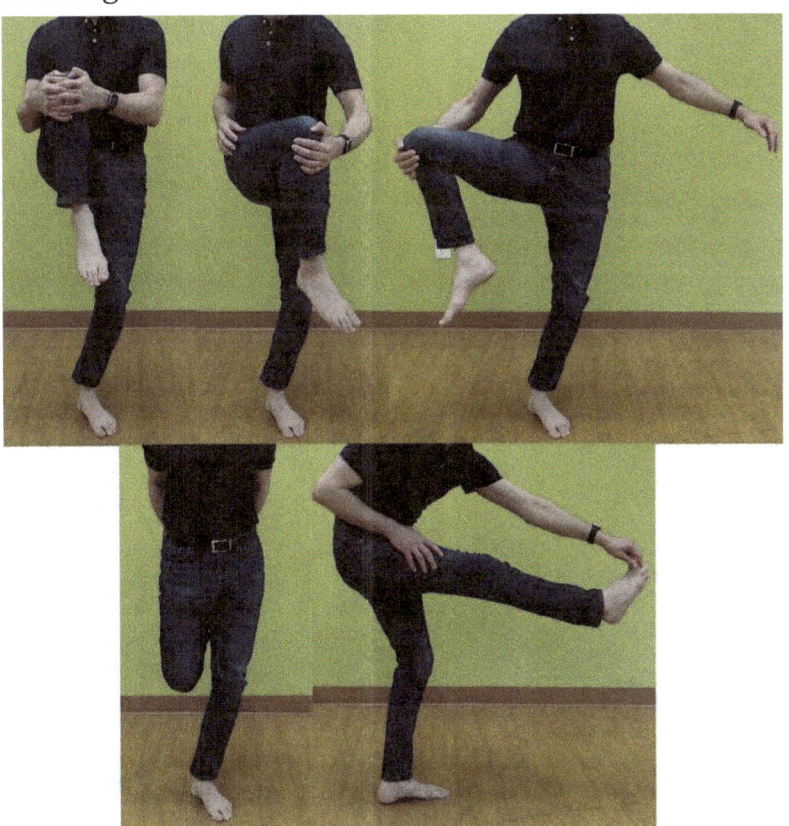

Figure 17: Stretching the leg up, in, out, back (or down), and forward.

Inner leg stretches: this is one of my favorite stretches, which I call the Spider-Man stretch. Start from a good posture (stand up straight!), then step out wide to your right with your right foot. Follow that leg down with your torso, bending your knee, until you can put your hand on the floor. At this point, your left leg should be completely straight. You can lift your left foot up so only your heel is touching the floor, if that helps. On your right leg, make sure your knee is directly above your toes, wherever they are pointed. If your knee is out of alignment with your toes, it can cause knee problems. Your foot can be up in the air (as in Figure 18) or flat on the ground. Each gives a slightly different feel. This should give you a good stretch on the inside of your left leg. When you're finished, move your feet under you and raise your head and body slowly so you don't get lightheaded. Repeat the whole stretch stepping out wide to the left with the left foot.

> I find it helpful to turn both the bent knee and toes toward a 45-degree angle from the original position. And if you need more of a stretch, you can press the elbow of your arm into the side of your bent leg to push it out farther.

This is a good introduction to static stretches, so let's go into dynamic stretches next.

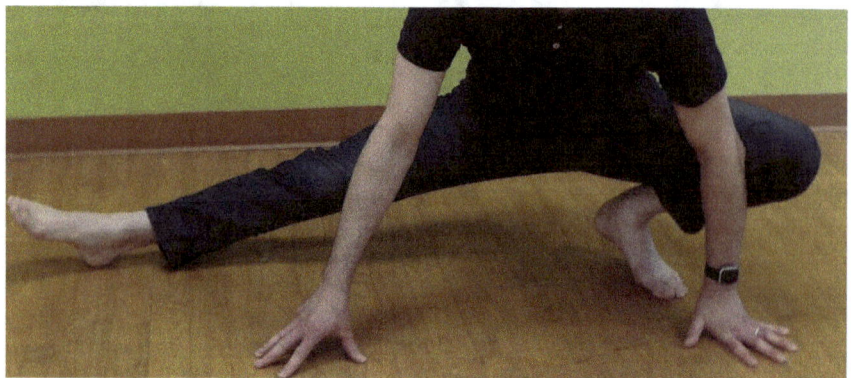

Figure 18: The "Spider-Man" stretch. Note the bent knee is in line with the toes.

Dynamic stretching

Dynamic stretching can produce a lot of the same results as static stretching, but in a shorter time. The drawback is that you must be careful not to hyperextend a joint (over stretch the joint in the direction it moves) while doing this. If you are double-jointed in your elbows or knees, pay special attention. It's best to start with a smaller range of motion and work up to the maximum range in which you feel comfortable. If it helps, keep a small amount of tension in the joints around the one you are stretching. If you've worked on the small muscles, this will be easier to do! For example, if you're moving your shoulder joint, keep your elbow a little tense so you don't flop around like a dead fish.

Here are some dynamic stretches I like.

Neck stretches: the neck is fairly susceptible to injury, and we'll cover this a lot in the section on not hurting yourself. For now, be careful when you do this. Don't go past your range of motion, don't jerk your neck, and don't try to move through two different directions at the same time. You'll learn why later on, but for now, trust me on this. First, as in the static stretch above, tilt your neck to one side (bringing your ear closer to your shoulder), pause for a moment when you get to your range of motion, then tilt to the other side so you don't strain your neck muscles.

You can also look straight up, then slowly bring your chin down to your left or right shoulder, then straight back up, then down to the other shoulder. These two stretches together should cover the range of motion of your neck.

Arm stretches: First make sure you have enough space around you. That's a whole arm's length in front, in back, side to side, and above you. Watch for hanging lights, kids, cats, and knick-knacks on tables!

Now, swing your arms forward, starting slow and moving a little faster if there's no pain or resistance. Reach all the way above your head when you do this. Full range of motion! Try to make your fingers touch in front of your face, then separate as they pass your waist. Make seven to ten circles. If you have shoulder pain or a rotator cuff injury, go slower on this, and I've found it helps if you keep your palms pointing away from your body (so your thumbs are pointing down), rather than inward (thumbs pointing up).

Next, reverse and swing both arms backward so your arms are coming up from hips to shoulders, then around in back of you. Try to touch your fingers as they rise in the front and keep your arms close to your head as they go around. Don't strain your shoulders to reach too far behind you. Also do this seven to ten times. After you get used to this maybe go up to fifteen revolutions, but you don't need to do more than that.

> This is another of my favorites, especially when standing up from sitting a long time, usually in front of a computer. When you type, you tend to keep the rest of your body rigid and your shoulders don't move.

Your arms should be feeling nice and loose at this point. Now you want to move your arms through their horizontal range of motion. Start with your arms extended straight out away from your sides, then come forward with both until your arms cross and your hands are hugging your opposite shoulder. Reverse direction and swing your arms behind you through their full range of motion, touching your hands together behind you, if you can. If it helps to find your range of motion, try to clap your hands together in front and touch your fingers behind you. If you have a large range of motion, you may be able to clap behind your back as well! Repeat this about ten times or so to really loosen the shoulder joints.

Torso stretches: while keeping your pants button or belt buckle facing forward, try to turn your shoulders from left to right and right to left. You should feel a line of tension reaching from shoulder to hip when you do so. This exercise can help to loosen up your lower back as well. Repeat about seven or eight times. You can twist a little harder on this one as you generally won't overextend anything here. Your back muscles are very dense and strong.

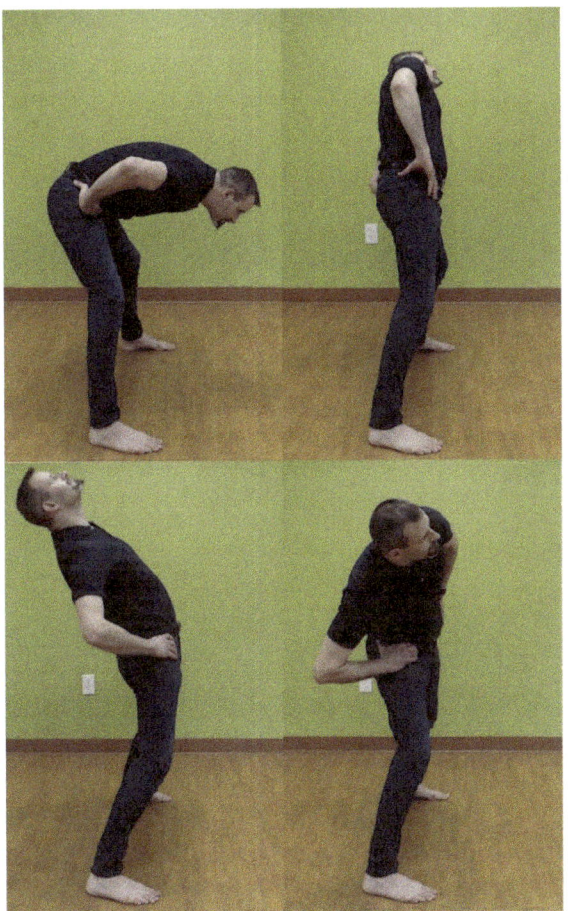

Figure 19: Hip stretches, moving circularly around the waist.

Hip stretches: This one is very nice for loosening your pelvis. Start from—what am I going to say? Yes, from a good standing posture—then bend forward so you can touch the ground with your fingers. If you can't touch the ground, move your feet out to a wider stance. Bend your knees for more balance. Then with your hands on your hips, circle your upper body, leaning to the left, behind you, to the right, and back to the front. Think of keeping your torso as low to the ground as possible while you go around in a circle. Take a very brief pause in the front. Repeat five times, then switch and rotate the other direction. As your hips become more limber, you will be able to circle your torso at a deeper angle.

Leg stretches: this one is very easy in theory, but make sure you don't lift your leg too high and strain your hamstrings. Use control and don't let the momentum of your swing determine how far your leg goes. Hold on to a chair, table, or wall if your balance is not the best. Start from a good posture (as always), feet under your hips, then lift (with controlled motion) one leg as far as it will go up in front of your face. Let your leg come back down, with gravity but controlled, to touch the floor with your toes about one and a half feet (half a meter) behind your starting position. Repeat eight to ten times with each leg. Try to engage your quadriceps and hamstrings when you do this, so you are pushing and pulling your leg up and down, rather than just swinging.

Knee stretches: bend at the hip and knees by about ten degrees and place your hands on your knees. Rotate your knees in small, slow circles, about the width of your foot. Your knees are not able to bend very far to the sides, but this circular motion will open up the joint. Repeat eight to ten times, both clockwise and counterclockwise. If you really want to, you can also do that move where you switch your hands over your knees, like your weird uncle does.

Ankle stretches: stand on one leg, making sure to bend your support knee (grab something for balance if needed!), and trace a circle with the toes of your raised foot. Go both clockwise and counterclockwise ten to twelve times. Stand on the other leg and repeat with the opposite foot. As an added bonus for this exercise, you can pair your hand motion to get a dynamic wrist stretch. While you have one foot in the air, trace a circle in the air with your fingers while you do the same with your foot. Go both directions with your foot and hand moving at the same speed. For an added *added* twist that will really break your brain, try going clockwise with your hand and counterclockwise with your foot, then vice versa! This one is good for flexibility, balance, and coordination.

Isometrics

Isometrics is the act of tightening your muscles without changing their length, both to warm up and to increase your flexibility. I'll give you a few exercises both for your arms and your legs, but you can also come up with others on your own. If you've never done this before, you may get a warm or buzzing feeling in the muscles you do this with. That's normal, and not, in fact, angry bees trying to escape your flesh.

> There are a lot more variations of dynamic stretching that you can experiment with. Just make sure you don't overextend your joints when you try them out. And remember that good posture! I bet you've already forgotten.

Leg stretches: to demonstrate how this works, we'll do the easiest version first. Start from a good posture—head back, shoulders back, hips tucked—and bend your knees slightly with your feet about the width of your shoulders, or a little bit wider. Plant your feet firmly on the floor, and starting with your thigh, pull inward with your entire leg, as if you want your feet and knees to come together. But don't let up the downward pressure on the floor! Your feet should stay in the same place. Tense your knee joint to protect it so it doesn't bend (like we did in the dynamic stretches), and try to pull your legs together with a fair bit of force.

Your legs may shake, and you may feel them grow warm. Still not bees. Hold this stance for a count of ten-one thousand. Now reverse, and while holding the same stance, keeping the muscles around your knees tense (which are more developed now you're doing squats, right?), push your feet apart, starting from the thighs. Again, your feet should not actually move. This time you'll feel the muscles on the outside of your legs engage and perhaps grow warm. Hold this for about ten seconds as well.

Come back to your good posture, this time with your feet about hip width apart, so narrower than before. Take a big step forward with one foot so your front knee is bent, and your back knee is mostly straight, though not locked out. Just like last time, tighten your muscles around your knees and don't let your feet or legs move. Then pull in as if you want both feet to slide directly under you. You'll feel the same stretch and warming sensation, this time on the fronts and backs of your thighs. Reverse this and push your front foot forward and back foot backward as if you are doing a split (but don't really do a split).

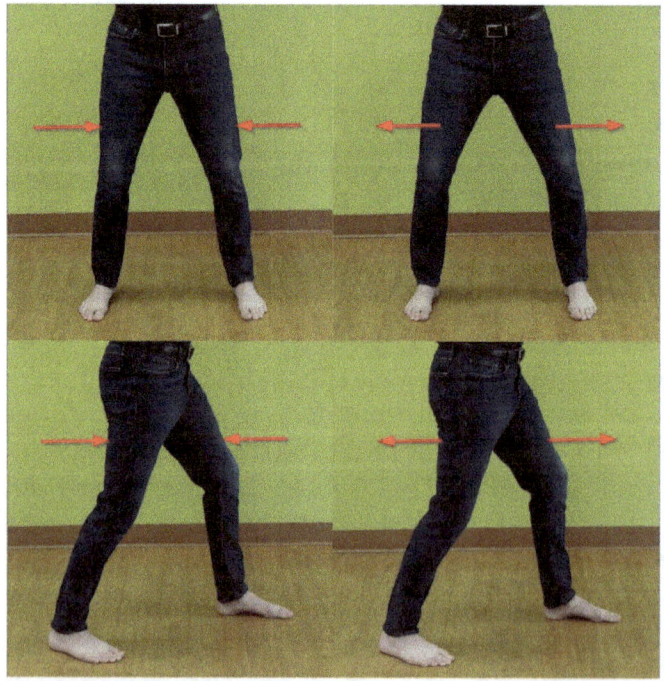

Figure 20: Isometrics, pulling in and pushing out standing with legs parallel (top) and after stepping forward (bottom). The force starts from the thighs.

Hold each position for about ten seconds. Next switch your legs so the other one is forward, and repeat both the pull in and the push out for about ten seconds. After this, your legs should be nice and warm, and your muscles should feel engaged.

Arm stretches: Let's try the same sort of exercises with your arms. You'll either press together as much as you can or pull away as much as you can. Here's the setup for your arms: put your hands together palm to palm with your fingers turned 90 degrees from each other so you can clasp your hands together. Have your elbows bent a little bit more than 90 degrees and push your hands together. Keep your shoulders down while you do this, because otherwise you can put too much stress on your shoulder joint. Then reverse and try to pull your hands away from each other while they're still clasped together. You may want to lower your arms a little bit to make sure your shoulders are not raising up. Hold both of these exercises for about ten seconds.

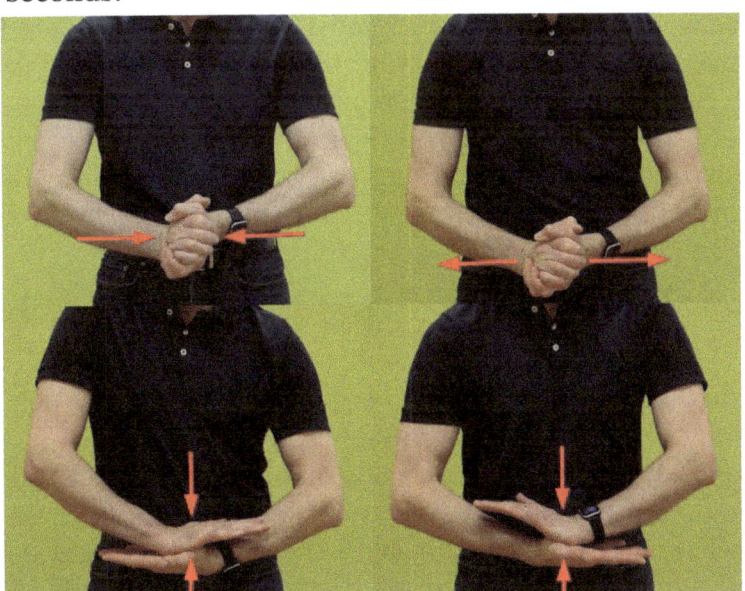

Figure 21: Isometrics, pushing in and pulling out (top) and pressing down with either hand (bottom).

For another variation, hold one hand just under your bellybutton, palm up, and close to your stomach, as if you're holding something up. Now put your other hand on top of the first one so the heels of both hands touch, and press both hands together. Don't let the muscles around your elbows and shoulders move, similar to what you did with your knees for the leg stretches. Keep your hands at about the level of your bellybutton while you do this. Remember to keep your shoulders low! Switch hands and do the same with the other hand on the bottom.

Those two exercises (pulling horizontally, then vertically) tend to get my arms feeling limbered up and warm. If you want some variations on this, you can put your palms and fingers together as in the first exercise, but this time keep your hands aligned so your fingers touch. With your fingers pointing upward, you can press your hands together and move slightly upward from your chest to about your chin, while pressing inward. Switch your hands so your fingers point down, you can do the same thing, pushing your arms inward, while moving from around your bellybutton to your hips. This one tends to work your chest muscles a little bit more, as well as the stabilization muscles in your shoulders.

Isometrics can be a great way to warm up when you're doing weight training, or if you're about to do hard exercise. These are also very nice if you've been sitting at a desk all day and your shoulders and legs are stiff. They can create the same effect as stretching out, but in a much smaller space.

Pandiculation!

Pandiculation is a fancy term for the involuntary stretching of the soft tissues, which you do while yawning. You know where you put both arms up above your head and sort of tense at the same time you reach your arms as far as they go? That's pandiculation. It's similar to the isometrics I talked about above, but rather than using two limbs in opposition to each other, you're tensing individual limbs.

The exact feeling is hard to describe, but it's sort of like pulling inward at the same time you're pushing outward.

It works as a kind of neural feedback loop to adjust how much tension you have in your muscles and put them back where they should be. Afterward, you may feel your shoulders, for example, falling into a relaxed position, especially if they've been up by your ears all day from dealing with stress. Because it's never easy to move when you're all tense, pandiculation also works to get you ready for activity.

> Pandiculation acts as a way to reset your neuromuscular system, especially if you've held the same position for a long time. If you've seen a cat or dog stretch after taking a nap, this is pandiculation.

Try it out yourself. Think about yawning, or read about yawning, or even just say yawning a lot. Yawning. Are you yawning yet? When you yawn, stretch your arms above your head and let them do what comes naturally. Do you feel the pandiculation function? If I'm sitting down, I like to continue the motion after stretching upward by putting my hands on my thighs and pressing downward. You can activate the same pandiculation response, and I find it often opens up my shoulders a lot (you might hear some pops and cracks!). Afterward, your arms will probably feel looser, as if you've just stretched them out.

You can do the same motion with your legs, for example if you stand up after sitting for a long time. Stand up and let the pandiculation response take over (yes, I like typing that word). I feel a tightening going from my knees, up through my upper thighs and into my butt. It feels similar to the isometric exercise where you're pulling your legs in toward each other. Afterward, continue the feeling by reversing direction and pushing out and down through your feet.

Observe when this happens naturally. Try to mimic the function voluntarily in your arms, or legs, or neck, or hips. This is similar to how I teach a lot of my martial arts classes. You can only teach somebody so much when breaking concepts down to their fundamental principles. At a certain point, you have to teach a person to observe themselves while they do an action, then let them copy and expand upon what they observe.

> Feel out the involuntary response that happens. Then learn how to channel it so if you feel stiff, you can pandiculate on command! But don't overdo it, as this function is still partially involuntary. You can mess up your joints if you do it too much or try to tense too much.

Add pandiculation to your stretching toolbox. The reason I give you so many types of stretches is because different stretches work better for different people. Try them all out and see what gives you the most benefit.

Stretching sequence

This is a sample of the stretching class I used to run at my day job once a week. This is geared for people who work primarily in an office, often sitting down for long periods hunched over a computer. There are a couple challenges if you're not used to complex motion or standing on one foot. If you do work in a desk-bound or sedentary job, this sequence of stretching may help you out as well. You don't have to restrict yourself to once a week either. If you do this every day you'll see a definite increase in your flexibility, and potentially a reduction in your

> You can find a video of this stretching sequence at:
> youtu.be/aniANeMQYio

tension or knots in your shoulders and back. Even running through this sequence two to three times a week will help. I usually go from the head down to the feet because it flows well for me. You don't have to do this, and can go from feet to head, or even just whatever feels best at the time. But try this stretching sequence as it's written a couple times to get used to it and see if it works for you. You'll notice this combines elements from both the static and dynamic stretching sequences, plus a couple extras.

Posture first! Fix your head, shoulders, hips, knees, and feet. I haven't harped on this in a while, but you should be used to doing it. You have been practicing, right? Using a timer to remind yourself? I'll assume you said yes. It's hard to hear through space and time.

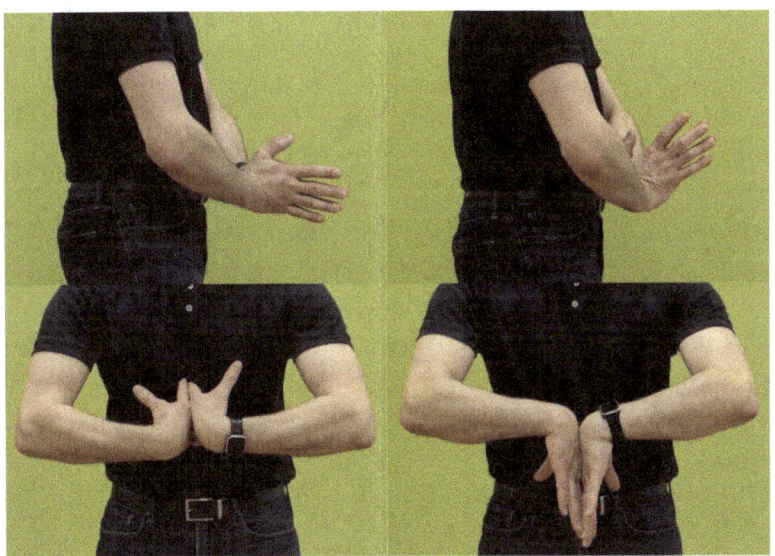

Figure 22: Wrist stretches with palms together (top) and backs of hands together (bottom).

Wrist stretch: This is good to loosen up your wrists if you've been using the computer and mouse for a while. You may hear a lot of popping and cracking in your wrists! First put your hands together, palm to palm, and press down and away from you to stretch your wrists (see the top two pictures in Figure 22). Your elbows will pop out from your sides, and you can wobble your hands back and forth to open your wrists up. Do this for about five seconds. Then switch so the backs of your hands are together, with your fingers pointing straight down. This time pull your arms upward and slightly away from your chest to stretch the other side of your wrists. Hold this for another five seconds, rolling the backs of your hands across each other.

Wrist, elbow, and shoulder rotations: Next, roll your wrists in circles through their full range of motion for eight to ten rotations. I like to go clockwise with my right hand and counterclockwise with my left to start so my hands are moving "outward." Then switch directions and roll the opposite way ("inward") for another eight to ten rotations. Keep your fingers loose while you do this. Now relax your wrists and move the rotation up to your elbows. Go outward and then inward in the same way, eight to ten rotations. Last, do the dynamic shoulder stretches described above, making big circles, using your full range of motion. Go forward, backward, then across your body. Make sure you have enough room and don't hit any furniture (or pets), including behind you!

Neck and torso stretches: Get into your good posture and expand upward as if your head is connected to the ceiling on a string, and the string is tightening. While keeping your eyes level (that is, don't look down or up), turn your head as far as it goes to the left. Hold this for a couple seconds, then turn your shoulders to the left as well, while making sure your knees are still in alignment with your toes. Hold for a few more seconds and feel the diagonal tension across your chest. Then repeat this sequence while looking to the right.

Next, continue with the static neck stretches described above, by looking up, then down. You can include some dynamic motion when you look up, by turning your chin side to side. Finally, do the static neck tilt, first to the left and then to the right, each for about ten seconds. Remember to reach your arm out to the side as if you can't quite reach something and drop your shoulders to get a good stretch in your neck tendons.

Torso twist: This is the same as the dynamic stretch above. Just keep your bellybutton facing forward and twist your shoulders until you feel a diagonal line of tension from shoulder to hip. Twist in both directions five to seven times.

Lower back stretch: This is a really good static stretch for opening your lower back, particularly if it aches. Simply lean forward and let your arms dangle to the floor. Your knees should be slightly bent. If you need to spread your legs out in order to touch the floor, that's fine. If your fingers are dangling in the air, that's fine too. What you want to focus on is letting the lower vertebrae in your spine release. Feel how, when you're bent over, your back slowly releases with the pull of gravity, since it's now going the opposite direction of how it's usually positioned (good upright posture, right?). The important part is to relax. If

A warning on this one: if this hurts a lot, don't do it! There may be something else wrong you need to get checked out. If you have a known back issue, clear this stretch with your doctor first.

you're very stiff, or if you have a known back injury, your back may hurt while you bend over. Try to feel where it hurts and see if relaxing that area lets you get closer to the floor. I'm talking here about "stiff" hurting, not sharp pains or continuous pain from injuries you know about. If you have a hard time relaxing, read through the next section, then come back to this one!

During this stretch, you should feel your spine lengthening, and your hands will gradually get closer to the floor. If you need more distance, bring your feet in some to let you stretch further. Hold this...well, really, hold it as long as you want. This is a position that benefits from the feedback of learning how to relax while you do it, which then lets you relax more, which then gives more feedback, and so on. Whenever you're done, come up SLOWLY, bending your knees as you roll up. You've just sent a lot of blood to your head while leaning over and if you come up too quickly, you may get tunnel vision or even fall over. It's best to "roll" up as if your back is a garage door that's opening up vertebrae by vertebrae until you're vertical (and in good posture!) once more.

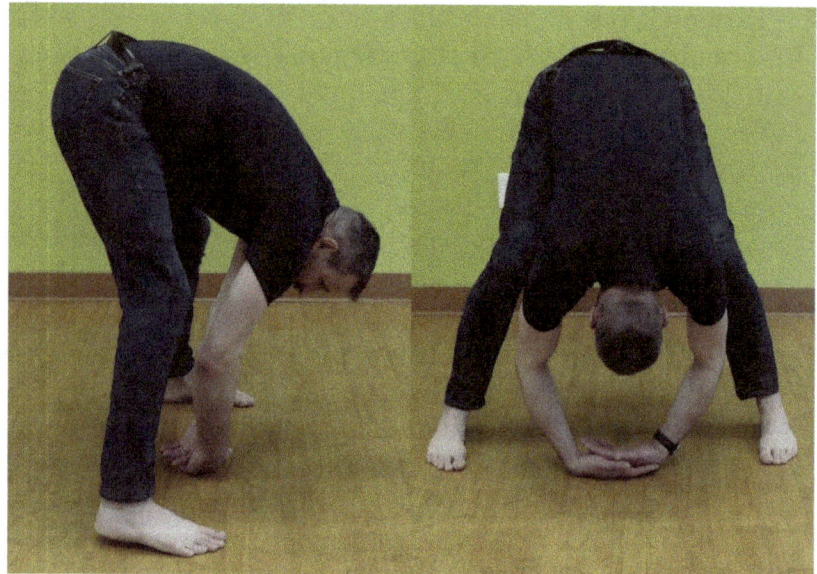

Figure 23: Lower back stretch. Make sure to relax into this position slowly over at least fifteen or twenty seconds.

Hip stretches: This is a good time to do the dynamic hip rotations from the previous section to loosen the connection between your upper and lower halves shown in Figure 19. Do five in each direction.

Leg stretches: From here on out, everything is about legs. The sequence I like to do is as follows. First do the static leg stretches, part one, from above (Figure 16: stepping out to the sides, first with your feet at 90-degree angles, then with your feet in line to the left and right).

Then do the static hip stretch (Figure 15), including putting your foot out in front for the foot raise and calf stretch. For a quick ankle stretch, get in good posture, and rock up to the balls of your feet, then back on your heels. Put your hands out in front if you need to, to keep your balance. Go from toes to heels seven or eight times.

Remember to use a chair, counter, or table for stability if you need to. These exercises give you a great chance to work on your balance!

Next do part two of the static leg stretches (Figure 17), lifting one foot at a time to stretch out your quadriceps and hamstrings. As an added ankle stretch, you can rotate the foot that's in the air around in circles, both clockwise and counterclockwise. If you feel really adventurous, add in hand rotations along with the foot rotations. If you go different directions with your hand and foot, it'll break your brain!

As an alternative, if you don't have a lot of time for leg stretches and do have a lot of space, you can do the dynamic leg raises to stretch both the quadriceps and hamstrings. Just be careful not to go too far and overextend, and also try not to kick anyone walking by...

Finally, do the static inner leg stretch, or "Spider-Man" stretch (Figure 18). Come back to the center after you do both sides and roll up again as you did for the lower back stretch.

Shake everything out. You'll feel nice and relaxed, and probably energized. Once you get used to this sequence, you should be able to do it in ten minutes or so. Doing it twice or three times a week will help your balance, flexibility, and coordination.

You're getting used to new muscle configurations. If you haven't done these types of stretches before, take it slow and let your body get used to it. Getting a massage or having a hot shower are good ways of getting tension out of your muscles while adjusting to more efficient movement.

Relaxing

We've talked about stretching out, but you should be able to relax, too. The biggest enemy of moving efficiently, or even using your body at all, is tense muscles. If you've ever seen professional fighters, or a gymnast, or a highly talented musician preparing to play, you may notice it looks like they're doing things effortlessly. That's because they are relaxed. They aren't fighting their own body.

An action—surprise!—is easier when your muscles aren't opposing that action. When you learn a skill and have repeated it so many times that it is innate, you "relax into it." You do this because you are not frightened or uncertain about what you're going to do. You've got this. It's easy.

Remember when you first learned to drive a car? Or if you don't drive, ride a bicycle? Or if you don't ride a bicycle, any other skill that takes a lot of time to master? The first time you do it, you're very uncertain and you don't know if it's going to go right in the end. You tense up. This makes it harder for you to learn as you don't know what you are doing, *and* you have to fight against your own muscles at the same time.

If you are tense in everyday motion, you add the energy required to tense your muscles to the amount of energy needed to perform that action. Let's reverse that trend. Your ideal state is to be completely relaxed when you're not actively doing something requiring muscles to engage. When you do need to use your muscles, there are some other tricks to give you an advantage. I'll cover those at the end of the book.

For right now, we're going to focus on simple relaxation. As before, let's start from the top. Stand, sit, or lie down. It doesn't really matter where you are. Actively focus on the top of your head. There are a lot of little muscles you don't think about that cover your skull. Now's the time to pay attention to them! The first challenge is to *be aware* that you can change the state of these muscles. When you're focusing on the top of your head, work to relax everything there. When it works, you'll feel a shift as the energy you're unconsciously holding in these muscles leaves, and they slide back to wherever gravity puts them.

After the top of your head, go down to your ears, and particularly your jaw. Pay attention to where your jaw meets the bottom of your ear all the way down to the bottom of your chin. Relax this whole system. Let the tension drain out. You may feel your jaw hanging open slightly. Often you just need someone to call attention to the tense area to realize it is tense. In fact, this area gets so tight that you can take another "pass" along it and relax more muscles the second time. Do this as many times as you need to feel all the tension in your jaw drain away.

Many people, especially when they are stressed, put a lot of tension into their jaw muscles. Unclench your jaw!

Once you lose the top layer of tension, you may feel another place you can relax, or you may immediately tense up again because your body is so used to doing so. Persuade your muscles it's alright to relax completely.

Your jaw is tied into your neck muscles, which are then tied into your shoulder muscles. The jaw is a huge lever that needs to be strong enough to tear through tough food. Thus, it's hinged nearly at the centerline of your skull. You may not realize it, but everything from your shoulders up to the top of your head is affected as you chew. So, if you are artificially keeping more tension in your jawline, that stress is reflected back into your neck, your shoulders, and your head. This is why you may get a headache when you're tensing your jaw. It's also why you may grind your teeth when you sleep while stressed.

Relax these muscles. I bet they've gotten tense again while you've been reading about tense muscles. I know mine have. This is often the first thing I notice if I am under pressure or have a deadline coming up. This is another good place to set a timer. This one might be as short as five seconds! Depending on how you deal with stress, you may clench your jaw tightly without even realizing it. In order to develop the habit of *not* tensing it, you must be aware of what's happening.

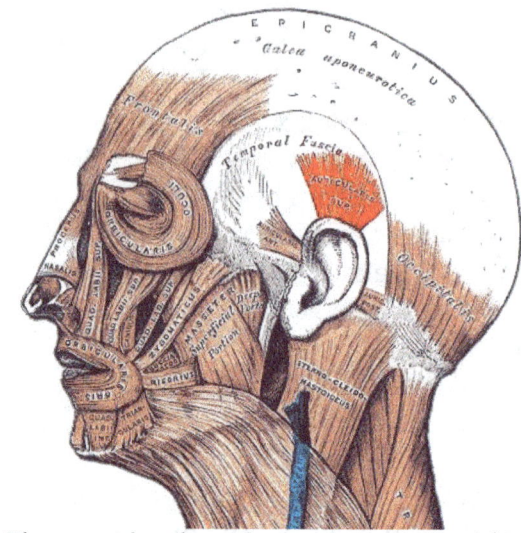

Figure 24: There are a lot of muscles to relax in the head (*Gray's Anatomy*)!

Now your jaw is relaxed (is it still relaxed?), let's keep moving down your body. Next is the shoulders. Remember the exercise from the beginning of the book? Up, back, and down. Or if you realize you're raising your shoulders up, simply let them fall. If you have your shoulders relaxed, it's a lot harder to tense up your back. Many back problems come from this combination of tense shoulders and tense jaw, because you're holding your upper body weird and— remember that bowling ball? If that weight is right above your center where it's supposed to be, then your back doesn't have to contort into a new shape to hold it upright. If you're hunched forward, tense, and tightening your jaw, you're making your back deal with a load extending forward.

Relaxing your lower back is another really good exercise, which I talked about last section in the stretching sequence. Now you're more aware of how to target individual muscles, try that stretch again and really pay attention to the muscles along your spine and in your lower back. Spend as much time as it takes to stretch out. If I do this, I'll basically end with my forearms horizontal and my elbows touching the floor after a bit of stretching.

The rest of your body tends to fall into line after you relax these parts. However, the other two areas that may be a problem are hands and feet. Remember to take breaks while you work to stretch them out. A really nice one is the wrist stretching exercise I detailed above in the stretching sequence, Figure 22.

> Especially if you do manual labor, or are on your feet a lot, your extremities can get tired, then try to compensate for the tiredness by tensing up.

Next, rotate your hands around the wrist in little circles. Switch and go the other direction too (this is also similar to the stretching sequence above). Curl your fingers in, then spread them wide. Repeat. Especially if you've been typing on a computer, you may hear a lot of little crackles in your wrists and hands as they open up.

You can also massage your hands. Hold your left hand out, palm up. Support the back of that hand with the fingers of your right hand. Now you can press your right thumb into the palm of the left hand. Especially concentrate on the pad below your thumb, and the web between your thumb and forefinger. Press—as hard as you're comfortable with—between the bones of your fingers, and also on the meaty pad below your pinky. Switch hands and do the same for the other one.

Obviously, this is hard to do with your feet, especially if you're wearing shoes, but the same actions apply. I can tell you, it feels really good to push a thumb right in the middle of your foot. You don't often get that feeling, especially if you wear shoes a lot.

Is your jaw tense again? How about your shoulders? I'm not being condescending here. This is also a reminder for me.

If you've gone to a yoga class, they often end in shavasana, lying with your back on the floor. You can practice this relaxation while doing that and run from your head to your feet. If you have trouble, it's relatively easy to find guided meditations online to aid in relaxation.

> Note for author:
> good posture,
> relax your jaw,
> untense your
> shoulders.

Add another note to the timer you set to maintain your good posture. You have done that, haven't you? When it goes off, reset your posture, then remember to relax as well.

Connection (Not the Opposite of Relaxing!)

The concept of connection is intertwined with relaxing, but is not the same thing, nor is it the opposite. To illustrate what I mean, let's use your hand as an example.

I like to think of your body as having three levels of tension. The first is completely relaxed. Hold your arm out and completely relax your hand. You may have to work at this because you're used to holding some tension in your hand. If it's completely relaxed, it's going to flop over the air and dangle from your wrist. If you shake your arm, your fingers will wobble around. This is completely relaxed, which is not actually very useful, unless you're lying down. If you completely relax your body, you collapse into a pile of limbs.

On the opposite end of the scale is complete tension. Don't do this for long, because it's not good for your joints and can cause cramps, but if you fully tense all the muscles in your hand, your hand is going to curl into a claw. Also not very useful, unless you're controlling the motion and turn your hand into a fist instead. This requires some other body mechanics, and a little bit of martial arts knowledge, so I'm not going to go into that here. For this example, and for general daily usage, you don't want to be fully tensed.

Last is what I like to call good connection. You use this a lot of the time, without realizing it. This is what you do when you are standing up but not doing any activity. What I want to teach you is to use the same good connection throughout all of your body rather than just portions. So for your hand, if you put your arm out in front of you, just holding your hand out "neutrally" is using a good connection in your hand. You're not letting it completely collapse, and you're not turning your hand into a claw. When you have a good connection, you can still move your fingers around and rotate your wrist, but there's just enough muscle usage to resist gravity. If you concentrate, you can feel a little tension to resist your hand fully collapsing. We're going to apply this concept to the rest of your body.

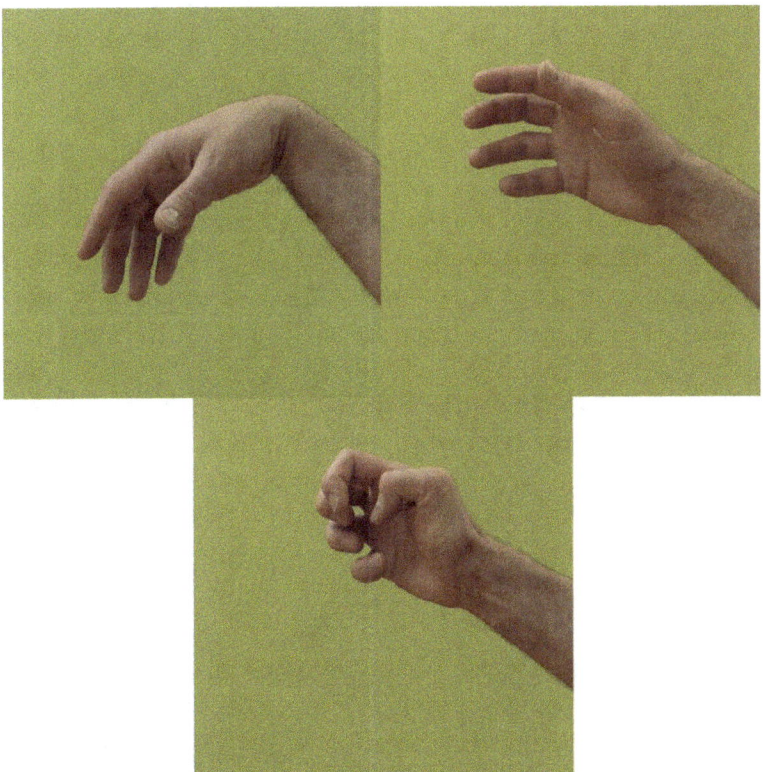

Figure 25: The hand fully relaxed, with connection, and fully tensed.

Again, get in your good posture. Head, shoulders, hips, knees. You will naturally be using a good connection for your legs, and if you put your hips and your shoulders in the right position, you should feel this tension in your abs as well. If you use a "lazy" posture as I described in the first chapter, with your shoulders slumped and your butt sticking out, this relaxes the muscles in the front of your body. That means you don't have to maintain a good connection with your abs, but your abs surround what? That's right, your center. So, it's beneficial to always have good connection in this part of your body. If you center is engaged, then you connect your hips to your shoulders, and it helps you stand or sit up straight.

Get in your good posture again (because you've probably slumped out of it while you've been reading, right?). The act of pulling your shoulders back and tucking your hips underneath you puts your abs in alignment. It should be easy to start feeling a good connection. If you can still relax your belly and let your stomach come out, try this: stretch your head up as if it suspended on a wire. When you do this, you're going to "expand" your body upward, and it is going to be very hard to keep your stomach relaxed. The reason I'm focusing on abs is because this is the main muscle that connects the lower half of your body—your legs—with the upper half of your body—your arms and head.

Let's try again. This time, relax, then put a hand on your belly. Loosen your abs. Now, while holding your hand on your stomach so you can feel the changes, get into a good posture. Feel how this affects your abs. Now expand upward, stretching so you feel your head connected to the ceiling by a wire. When you do this, your abs should stretch out even more and you'll be forced to maintain a good connection between your hips and your shoulders. While keeping everything else in place, just try to relax your abs. It's pretty hard! We'll play around with this after covering anatomy.

Here's one last quick exercise to show you why keeping a good connection in your abs is helpful. First, we'll do the relaxed situation. Shake out your body and go back to your regular stance, whether your shoulders are rounded, butt is out or whatever. Twist your shoulders from side to side, then bend to your left and bend to your right. Your hips don't have to move while you do this, do they?

One last time (for right now), get in a good position, tuck your hips as in Figure 4, and expand upward. Feel the connection of your abs between your hips and your shoulders. Now do the same exercise: twist your shoulders and try to bend to your left and right. You should feel your hips start to come along with the motion. This is because you've now connected your hips to your shoulders, and that is what I mean by connection rather than relaxation.

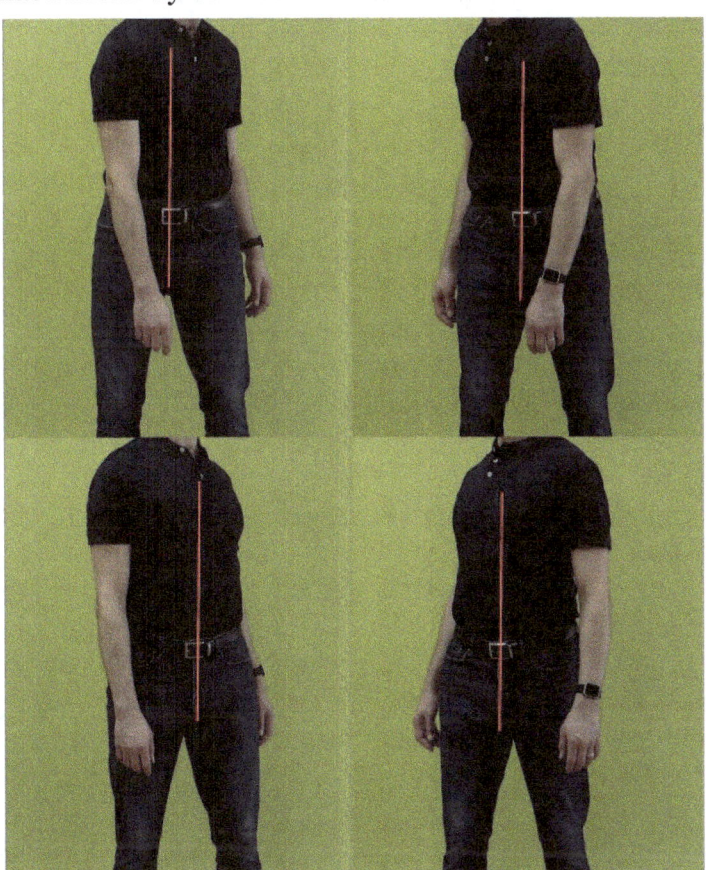

Figure 26: Note the hips don't move when twisting with little connection. With good posture and connection, the hips start turning with the motion.

Remember how this feels, because after we go over some basic anatomy, we're going to put these concepts together into how to walk, and how to use your arms. But, we're coming at this from first principles, as if you're completely new to this body you have. You (hopefully) understand by now how to keep yourself limber and relaxed, with good posture.

"Interior" and "Exterior" muscle

A final topic before we get to anatomy. Time to dig into something not well understood in the medical community, even in the last few years. This is the difference between "exterior" muscles—the ones we talk about most of the time, like your biceps, quadriceps, and deltoid muscles—and "interior" muscles, which is comprised of your small muscles and fascia.

What's fascia? You might have heard about it if you watch medical TV shows as something a surgeon will cut through to get to larger muscles or organs. It's the bands of thin muscle that connects muscles and organs to each other. It's the muscle for your muscle. Fascia has traditionally been thought of as passive tissue, just transmitting tension through the larger muscles and supporting nerves and blood vessels. But, you can actually manipulate your fascia, similar to your larger muscles. It just takes a bit more effort because you don't usually do so.

Let's take the abdominal muscle as an example. One of the examples I use is the rectus abdominis. Fascia is all over your core, binding together the muscles that make up the "six-pack" on your belly. You can tighten your whole core at once, right? It's what you do when you pull your gut in to impress someone. But you can move this fascia around in different ways, tightening, loosening, and even shifting larger muscles to some degree. It's a fascinating subject, and we're going to dig into it in the "core" and "back" section of anatomy. For now, keep it in mind, and maybe play around with moving your fascia. Here's a couple other examples.

There is a ton of fascia surrounding your head and neck. A lot of times, this is what's tensing up when your jaw or neck is tight. Pay attention to your jaw, and first relax the big muscle, so you're not gritting your teeth. Now, try to relax everything surrounding your jaw. This sort of feels like a warmth or tingling spreading from your cheeks to your ears. It takes a little concentration to do this, so you may not get it on the first try or might need to relax several times in a row.

You can do the same thing with your neck. Find a neutral position (one with good posture, yes?), then find that same release of warmth or tingling across the back of your neck. For a harder challenge, try activating the fascia down your forearm or across the back of your shoulder.

This will be *really* helpful for exercises toward the end of this book, so now when I talk about "interior" muscle, you'll know what I mean. When you strengthen the little muscles and support muscles in the wall push-up and squat exercises above, that's also training your interior muscles to help your external muscles do their jobs.

Anatomy

A quick note on how to use this section. There's a *lot* going on here with respect to anatomy, and it's very important to at least be familiar with how your body is put together. That said, there's also a lot of description here. The book after this point will be broken up into descriptions of actions with the lower body, the upper body, then the whole body. So if you find your eyes starting to glaze over despite my best efforts to entertain you, I might suggest reading the section on leg anatomy, then taking a break and reading the section on how to walk. After you've absorbed that, then come back to the anatomy of the arms, and read the accompanying section. Alternately, you could read this all the way through and refer back to individual anatomy sections as you need. Or you could even read this back to front for some reason! You do you.

Anatomy of the Lower Body

This next section details the anatomy from your feet up to your core. I won't be naming muscles (mostly), but I will be going through some of the kinematic connections and how your lower limbs are supposed to work. Please don't skip this part, even if you read it out of order. Paying attention to how your body is connected is one of the major steps in learning how to operate it. I promise I'll make this as exciting as possible.

Feet and Ankles

I bet you think about your hands a lot, since you use them every day for all sorts of activities. However, how often do you think about your feet in the same way? They are equivalent to your hands in many respects, although you put more weight on them, and they are specialized for the action of walking rather than grasping and manipulating. That said, they can still do a lot of the same things, and you can use your hands as an example of how to learn to operate your feet better. For this section, if you have the freedom to, take off any shoes and socks, and let your bare feet contact the floor. This will help you feel what I'm talking about.

After the anatomy section we'll review the action of walking, but for now, place your feet flush to the floor, then try to feel where your foot contacts the ground. If you have flat arches, this may be nearly the entirety of the bottom of your foot. If you have regular or high arches, your foot may only contact along a "C" shape going from the pads of your foot to your heel. Then there are those stubby things at the end of your feet. What are toes for anyway? They don't have the same manipulative power as your fingers do, but they still play a big part in your balance.

Move your feet through their whole range of motion. Stand on one foot, lift the other up, waggle your toes, and roll your ankle around as in the stretching sequence I covered in the previous section. You have a bunch of joints in your foot—just as many as you do in your hand. We'll cover them in the section on hand anatomy. For your feet, these can be incredibly helpful for walking. They also help you balance. Stand up straight with good posture (as usual) and try to move your balance around with just your feet. Can you push off with your toes so much that you start to tip backward? Can you pull with your toes and go forward?

Can you lift your toes up while you leave the rest of your foot on the ground? Can you move your toes individually? If not, it's likely because you've never practiced. This is why it's important to explore your anatomy (and yes, I know how that sounds...). You may be able to do things you never thought you could, just because you've never tried.

Rock up to the balls of your feet and back to your heels as in the stretching section, but this time, feel how your toes react.

There's another axis of rotation for your feet which people often disregard, and that is side to side. Try rolling to the outsides of your feet so you're just standing on the "ridge edge" of your foot. Let your knees push outward as well, so they are still above your feet. If you can hold this position, you may find that it's actually more stable for balance than standing flat on your feet. Ha ha! I've tricked you into something I'm only going to explain in more detail near the end of the book. Now you're going to have to keep reading!

> If you stand for long periods of time, or your Achilles tendon is tight or weak, then you run the risk of inflaming the plantar fascia (that connective strip). Moving your feet around, wiggling your toes, and rolling side to side will help.

For now, let's move on to the next joint.

The Achilles Tendon

The Achilles tendon is vital to walking. We found it before, in the section on muscles, tendons, and ligaments at the beginning of the book. I hope yours is still in the same place.

I'll give you one really good exercise for your Achilles tendon. This also has the added benefit of helping to prevent plantar fasciitis (the inflammation of the strip of connective tissue on the bottom of your feet between your heel and your toes).

This one is pretty easy. Just stand with good posture and bring your center slightly forward so that it's over your toes rather than over your heels. As you do this, you will naturally start to raise your heels, just like the exercises with your center from the first chapter. Use this motion, with your weight over your toes, and push upward, extending. Hold for about five seconds, then put your heels back on the ground. You can exercise your Achilles tendon by doing these heel raises. It's easy to do while you're standing somewhere, for instance brushing your teeth. Just come up to your toes, then back down to the ground. You can also find a ledge (for example, a stair close to ground level) so that rather than coming back to ground, you can flex until your heels are lower than your toes. Be certain of your balance and don't fall! This will give an added dimension to help stretch out the fascia on the bottom of your foot. You'll also feel this lengthen your Achilles tendon and exercise your calf muscle.

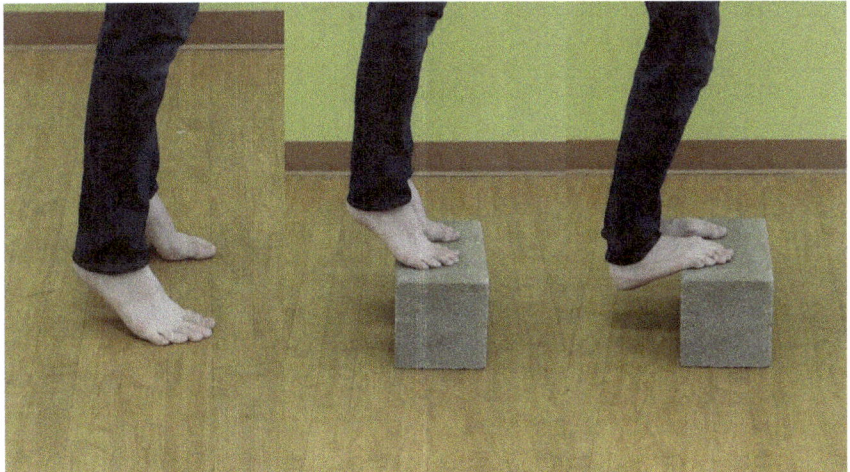

Figure 27: Calf raises on the floor (left) and on a ledge (right).

See if you can hold this stretch for a few seconds before you come back down. As you get better, try to extend the total time you can stand on your toes. Try for ten seconds. If you can do that, then go for longer. If you do this every day, add a second or two each time you do it. Soon you will be able to stand on your toes for longer periods of time. This is also really useful if you're trying to reach something up on a high shelf!

As a final challenge, once you get proficient at this, come up to standing on your toes and the pads of your feet only.

Hold this. Walk around on your toes. If you are used to high heels, this may be pretty easy. If you're not, this is a great calf-building exercise. Plus, it's just cool to do.

Knees

Let's talk about your knees. Specifically, the relationship between your knees and toes. I often get on my martial arts students about this, because if you bend your knees wrong a lot, you can mess up the knee joint over time. Then you're due for a knee replacement later in life, which is a big hassle and a lot of pain. Avoiding it with proper posture and movement is easier, less painful, and will save you a lot of money.

First sit down in a chair. Remember your good posture! Your shoulders should be back, your head above your center, and your feet out in front of you. In this position, your knees should be directly above the center of your feet. This is generally where you want to have them whatever you're doing. Now stand up. Again, your knees should be above your feet. This is the orientation you should keep for almost everything you do.

Try this exercise briefly while standing, but don't leave your knees in this position: Keep your feet steady on the floor, toes pointing straight forward, but start bringing your knees in as if you are going to make them touch. Do you feel that stretch or strain on the outside of your legs? You may also feel some tension on the side of your knee facing your other leg. Go back to your starting position, knees over toes. Do the same thing but outward. If you push your knees outward, then you should feel the opposite strain on the inside of your calf and on the side of your knee facing out from your body. Come back to center. If you try to put your knees in these positions while you do any sort of activity, that tightness that you felt will be magnified, and can lead to straining or rupturing ligaments or tendons. This is what happens if you step wrong and roll your ankle, for example.

If your knees aren't straight, the weight on your feet is not going straight up (or down) your leg. Instead, it's going to the side of your leg, away from the powerful muscles in the middle and into the smaller, more fragile supporting muscles on the outsides of your knees. If you are holding a heavy object or doing some activity, the load on your feet can go up by a significant fraction of your body weight.

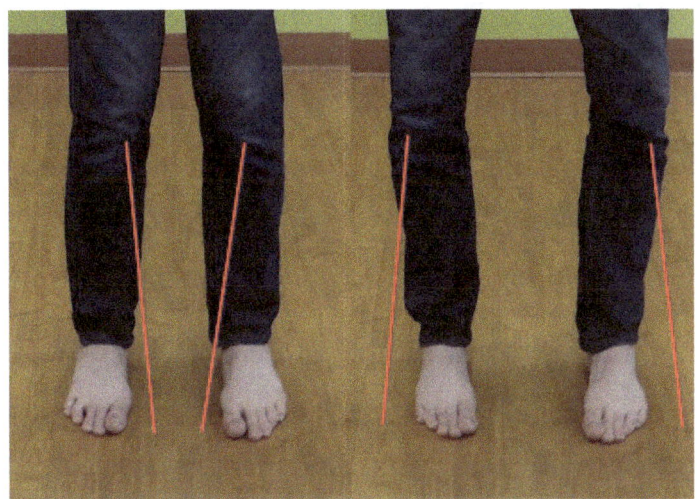

Figure 28: Your knees should line up with your toes. Here the knees are not lined up, causing excess stress.

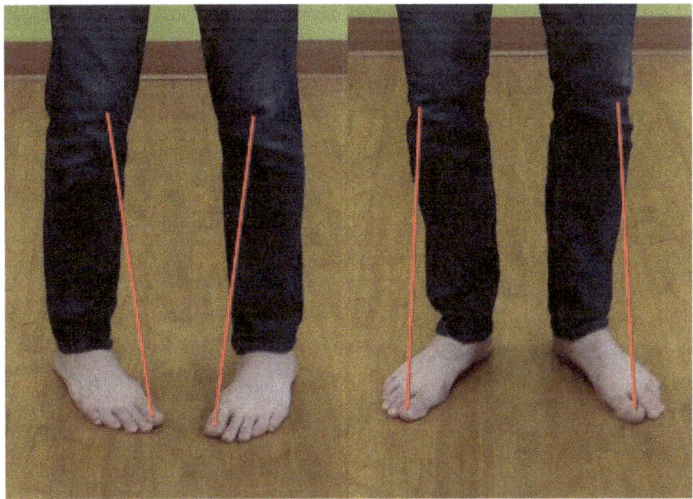

Figure 29: Here the knees are aligned with the toes.

When you walk, you should not let your knees drift to the inside or outside of your feet. Even if you bend your knees, or squat down, your knees should stay in line with your toes.

Note: your feet can rotate quite a bit! Your knees should follow them. So if, while standing, you turn your toes in toward each other, your knees should be facing inward, right above them. The same thing should happen if you turn your feet out forty-five degrees, so you make a large pizza wedge. Your knees should also now be pointing out forty-five degrees to each side—above your feet. If your knees don't follow your toes, you'll get the same stress as described above and potentially cause damage to the knee joint.

Knees and elbows—whose connective roles are similar—are two of the joints that take the most abuse in daily action. Done correctly, an exercise to help combat degradation and injury in your knees is squats (spoilers—the one for your elbows is wall or regular pushups). Often the subject is met with a groan as it's not popular like bench presses or leg lifts, but I'm going to spend some time talking about them because they're very important for good leg health.

Let's go through the process of a good squat. I described a squat on a wall in the muscles section. If you've mastered that, this is the next step. First, get in a good posture with your feet about your shoulder or hip-width apart. Second, I want you to start the motion with (surprise!) your hips. Because they're tucked under you (they are tucked under you, aren't they?), you can reverse that and start to stick your butt out. If you did the example showing how to move your center, then

> Your eventual goal is to get your butt almost to the floor, but it's perfectly fine to start with squatting only a few degrees, then slowly increase your squat until you get your thighs horizontal. If you need to, hold onto a tabletop or counter with your hands while you do this to make sure you don't fall backward.

you know you'll feel like you're starting to fall backward. This is what you want to feel in this instance. You can put your arms out in front of you to help with the change in your center of mass. Try to get your center over your heels rather than over the center of your feet. This is going to force you to work on the correct muscles for a good squat.

Start bending your knees more and more, making sure to keep them over your feet, and don't let them drift to either side. Go down as far as you are able, keeping your hands out in front to help your balance. You should feel like you're almost falling backward the whole way down. Keep your

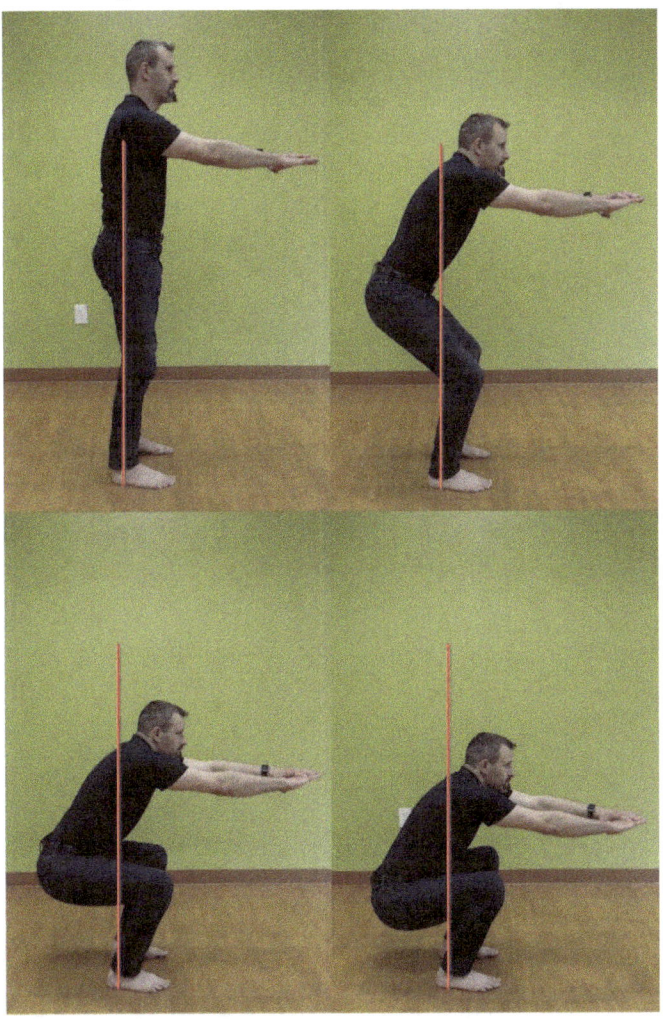

Figure 30: The stages of a squat. Notice the center of mass (red line) stays above the heels.

torso upright, and don't give in to the urge to lean forward—that will put your weight over your toes, which will both defeat the purpose of the squat and put your knees under more stress. Come back up—slowly in the same manner—still with an upright torso. Finish in a good posture.

If you're keeping your weight on your heels, you might have to step back and catch yourself sometimes. This is fine! After getting used to going down to where your thighs are horizontal (as shown in the lower left in Figure 30), work your way down until you can just about sit on the floor.

Do the squat very slowly for best effect. Once you understand your balance while moving, try it without holding on to anything. You'll use your leg muscles more!

Feel all the little muscles that are engaging around your knees while you perform a squat. These little muscles are what you're going to build if you do the squat in a slow and controlled manner, rather than doing it quickly. All those little muscles, when they are built up, help keep your knees centered and over your feet, even when you're not thinking about it.

The key to squats is to start small. The best starting place is probably the squats with your back against the wall, just to make sure you don't injure your knees, which is the whole point of this. Try to do ten of those a day for a week and see if your knees feel stronger. Keep either adding more squats or going lower slowly and steadily, and you'll be surprised what you can do!

If you have trouble doing squats, here's an alternate way to get started. While in good posture, place your heels about a foot and a half away from a wall. As in the wall squats, start sticking your butt out until you can rest against the wall. Now use the wall as a support so you can move up and down in a good squat. You may not need to use your hands as a counterbalance in this case.

However you do your squats, making it a daily routine to do at least five or ten can be incredibly beneficial in building up your knees over a period of a month or so. If you want a challenge, try to work up to thirty squats every day, and do it over a month. You can also change up how deep your squats are. See if you can get your butt all the way to the ground, then back up to full standing position. As you get better at this you can move your feet closer together to give you even more of a challenge.

Thighs

Your quadriceps (in the front of your leg) and hamstrings (back of leg) are the equivalent of your biceps (top of your arm) and triceps (bottom of arm) in your upper body. But the muscles in your legs are generally much larger than the ones in your arms. They are the powerhouse of your body, along with your core muscles. The squats I described above will help you develop these muscles, along with the small stabilization muscles around your knees.

But while your quadriceps and hamstrings are very powerful, it's always important to look at the connections at the ends of the muscles. These are often referred to as muscle "heads." A powerful crane is only as good as the foundation it's built on. If you can lift 100 pounds (or 45 kg for you metric types), but the connection between your quadriceps and your knee can only support 90 pounds (fewer kg...) then what happens? Your crane crushes its base. Except instead of a base, it's your knees. Muscle heads usually connect near a joint, and joint problems are one of the hardest things to repair or heal.

Let's look at the end of your thighs near the knees first. They are one of your most exposed joints, along with your elbows. Take a seat and let's go through some of the muscle connections. Put a hand on your knee and let your fingers trace where the tendons join to the kneecap. We're going to go through those connections, then to their other end, where the tendons disappear into the large muscle of your quadriceps.

Keep your hand on your knee and slowly stand up from where you're seated. You should feel the muscles on the sides of your knees retract, or move out of the way, while the tendon connecting the top of your kneecap to your quadriceps gets very tense, then relaxes when you fully stand up. There are a whole bunch of little connections here, and if any one of them gets damaged, the rest of them have to take over to help. The more you can protect and strengthen these tendons the better.

Let's try this again with the underside of your knee. Sit back down, then put both hands on one of your knees so that your thumbs are on the top of your leg and your fingers wrap around underneath your knee. You should feel several large ropey tendons on the underside of your leg connecting your lower leg to your upper leg. If you explore very carefully, you should feel two on the inside and one on the outside. Sit all the way straight back in a good posture. Now, while lightly gripping your leg, I want you to stand up. Feel those tendons shift around? If, for example, you're feeling your right knee, and you lean very slightly to your left as you stand, you may feel the tendons on the interior of the underside jerk before you stand up. These are the tendons of your hamstrings activating to pull your body forward so that you can stand. You can feel the same sort of thing if you stand on one leg (with a bent knee), and open and close the leg that you have in the air with your hand underneath your knee. You'll feel those tendons go taut, then relax.

I find the motion of the kneecap one of the most interesting in the body. Your mileage may vary.

This is sort of like the hinge of your leg. You know those metal doohickies on the top of screen doors? When you open the door, they extend and slowly retract back to close the door. This is a similar action to what's going on with the tendons underneath your knee.

They provide a lot of explosive power to your movement, especially with things like running or jumping.

Now, since you're feeling yourself up, move your hand through the lower portion of your thigh, even to that ridge underneath your butt. Try the same exercise: sitting down and standing up while feeling this area. You may need to use both hands because this muscle is much larger than your knee. Along with the major contraction and expansion of muscles you may also feel something like hard ridges that suddenly pop up, then disappear, especially on the inside fold between your quadriceps and your belly. This is similar to what's happening in your knee. You're feeling the tendons go rigid in order to pull your muscles quickly to a new position. This, in turn, pulls your bones where you want them to be.

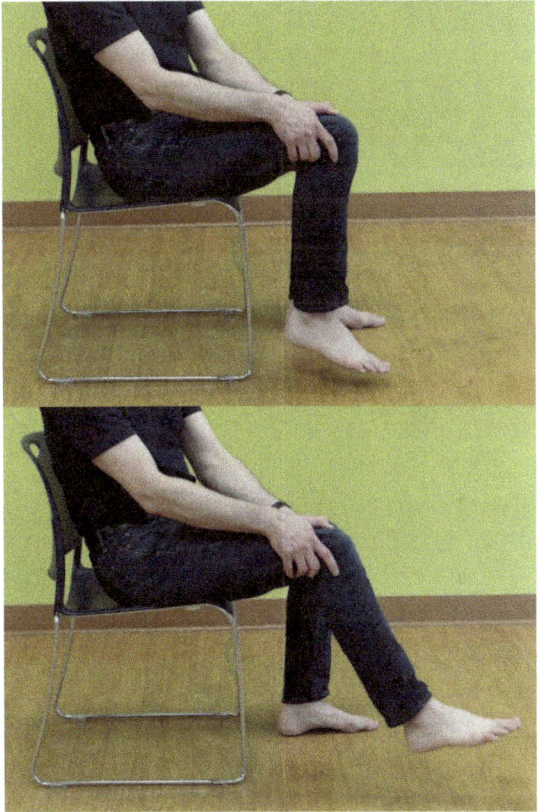

Figure 31: Feel the tendons under your knee to better understand how your thigh muscles work.

Okay, now that we've talked about the ends of your thigh muscles, let's talk about the muscles themselves. First, the quadriceps (the ones in the front of your leg). These muscles act in opposition to your hamstrings, just like your biceps and triceps act in opposition to each other. This enables you to move your leg (or your arm) in very quick motion because you can pull on both sides of the bone in quick succession, thus moving it very fast. The quadriceps is the muscle group that has four connections, or "heads" reaching all around your kneecap. The other end attaches up into your pelvic bone. You can feel this if you put your finger right where your hip bends, then lean over a little bit. You'll feel a hollow appear as the muscle contracts and expands.

> There are a lot of little stabilization muscles around the joint of your hip and if they weaken, or if any of them tear, then the rest have to take over for them. That increases the wear on the hip joint, and you're on the road to eventual hip replacement!

Interestingly, the large head of the quad that makes up that impressive bulge on gymnasts, swimmers, and other athletes (the rectus femoris, seen in Figure 32), is actually pretty weak in helping you stand up and in extending your knee. The other three heads of the muscle do more, because they connect to the sides of your knee and help stabilize the entire compound muscle on the front of your thigh.

The hamstrings work in opposition to the quadriceps, but only some of the time. Try this exercise: put one hand on the front of your thigh (the quadriceps) and the other hand on underside of your thigh (the hamstrings). Do the same exercise of going from a standing position (in good posture, right?) to a seated position.

You can feel how both muscles pull on your leg bones while they support your body in motion. However, they activate at different times with the quadriceps working a little harder while you sit down and the hamstrings working a little harder when you stand back up. You can also feel a difference while walking. Put one hand on top and one hand on bottom of your thigh again, then take a step with the *opposite* foot. You'll feel the quadriceps relax a little bit as the other foot goes forward and the hamstrings tighten. Then as you pull that foot forward to take the next step, you'll feel the quadriceps start the movement. This pushing and pulling motion is the majority of how we walk and is tied directly to your hips. You didn't think I'd forgotten about your hips, did you? The push/pull motion is very useful in the mechanisms of walking, but for now, let's move onward and upward. We can't round out the topic without talking about how your legs connect to the rest of your body.

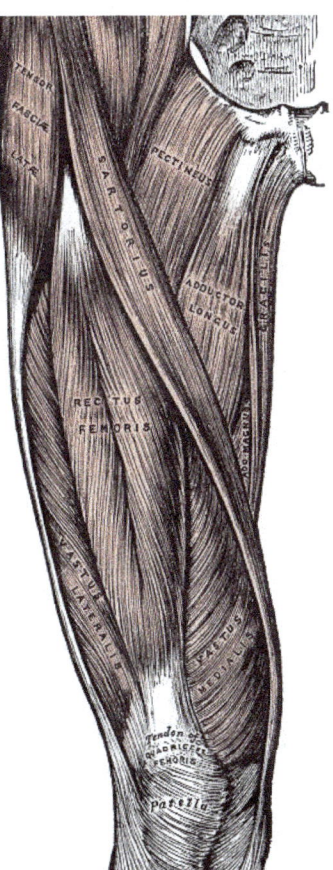

Figure 32: The muscles of the thigh (Gray's Anatomy).

Hips

The hips. I can talk about these joints for a long time. I've taught several martial arts classes focusing almost exclusively on the hips and how they move. They are the equivalent of your shoulders for your lower body, but unlike your shoulders, they support your weight all the time. Thus, for things like posture, lower back support, walking, and even sitting at a computer, your hips are very important, and you shouldn't forget about them.

Let's try a similar exercise to the one in the previous section. Put your hands on your hips with your palm right on the edge of your pelvic ridge (which should be the thing holding your pants up on the left and right of your waist), your thumb going forward around the circumference of your hips, and your fingers trailing down into where your quadriceps meets your butt. Now walk.

Okay, wait, come back. Did you remember your posture? Fix it.

And take this book with you.

> I've been talking about the hip area for the whole book. Yes really. Go back and look if you don't believe me. Posture: tuck your hips. Center of mass: this is where your hips are. Stretching: contains both a static and dynamic hip stretch. Hopefully you're starting to realize how important these joints are. It's what joins your legs to the reason you have legs.

Okay, now walk.

The first time, walk about ten steps with your hips in the "lazy" position, with your belt buckle pointing downward. Then turn around and walk back to where you started. Next walk back and forth with your hips tucked like I told you in the section on posture. You feel all those little connections and moving tendons and muscles in your hips? These are all the connections that keep you upright, and let you walk. And...I actually can't go into this in as much detail as I want right now, because I haven't taught you how to walk yet, and we haven't gotten to the really juicy bits yet. For now, remember how all those little connections felt underneath your hands. Go for a long walk and just feel how all the little muscles wrap around your hips and activate as you move your legs. Stand still and shift your hips around in a little circle. See which muscles activate while you do that. A lot of this you're going to have to feel for yourself. Keep in mind what I've gone over with your quadriceps, hamstrings, and hips. There will be a test later.

This is also a good place to address differences in body shape. For example, bodies with more estrogen express more female characteristics and bodies with more testosterone express more male characteristics. That's a very simplistic way of looking at it, but this also affects hips. Estrogen can widen the hips, increase fat stores around the hips and thighs, and potentially loosen ligament connections. In practice, this means the way the hips move might be at a slightly different angle. In my martial arts class, we're actively working on how some of the traditional movements—in the past only taught to men—don't work as well for women. We don't have a full assessment, but this is worth thinking about as you go through the section on walking, especially if a movement doesn't feel quite right.

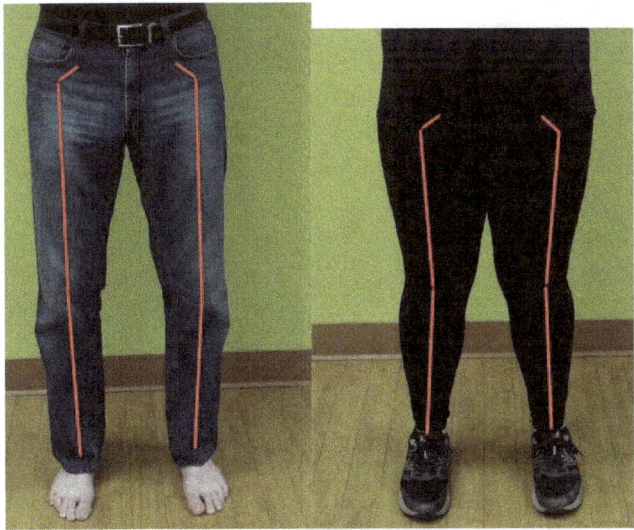

Figure 33: Note the difference in how the hips connect with wider and narrower hips. This affects walking gait.

Glutes

You knew this was coming, didn't you? You're going to feel your own butt. Put one hand on each of those glorious glutes and take another walk. You can leave the book here for this one. Just remember your posture and keep your head up and your hips tucked. Make this walk a little bit longer. Try to walk around objects, or turn corners, or lean forward and backward.

Go on, I'll wait here.

Are you back? Did you feel all the connections and the different muscles activating as you moved? Obviously, a lot of this overlaps with your hips, since they are connected to your butt. Different parts of your glutes trigger as you take steps and move in different directions. Keep these connections in mind when I teach you how to walk. For now, I'll give you an overview of the structure of your gluteus. Think of this as Hips: Part Two. This is the all-important area of connection between your lower and upper half.

Your butt is made up of three main muscles: the gluteus maximus, medius, and minimus. Most of what you feel is in the maximus muscle. In contrast, some of the upper connections when you were feeling your hips was the gluteus medius. Most of the minimus is hidden underneath the medius, which—like the little stabilization muscles in your knees and shoulders—mostly helps you keep your hips level as you walk. The whole gluteus collection of muscles is specific to humans because we are the only animals who walk completely upright. It can help you stand up for long periods of time, especially if you use good posture. Were you wondering if I was going to bring posture up again?

While the gluteus muscles help you stand up, if you sit down for long periods of time—for example if you are in an office job—the gluteus can weaken. You want to make sure you take care of it. One good method is the squats I described near the beginning of the book, and again in the section on your thighs. Try a squat with your hands on your butt and see how the muscles change shape!

Without such strong muscles keeping us upright, we would start to bend forward like an animal walking on all fours. Tucking your hips engages your glutes, which also engages your thighs, enhancing your posture. Now you've got a little experience holding on to your butt as you walk, you'll be able to feel the difference when you walk efficiently rather than walking, well, like you usually do. Stay tuned!

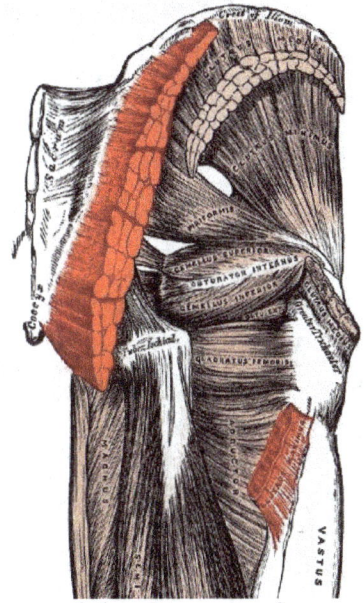

Figure 34: A cutaway of the gluteus muscle group (Gray's Anatomy). The maximus is cut away (highlighted), as is the medius.

Core

This section of your body could probably have its own book, and we'll discuss the core in the section on legs, on arms, and then again in some applications at the end! As your hips are the connection between your lower and upper half, your core contains the muscle that lets you activate it. By no coincidence, this is also where your center of mass resides. Remember how I said if you control the center of mass of something, you control how it moves? Your core muscles can help make the difference in graceful, efficient movement, and lazy, slow movement.

Another concept many fitness guides don't cover is that the muscles in your back are just as important as the ones in your abdomen. If you've got really developed abs, but haven't worked on any of the musculature of your lower back, you're more likely to slump forward, and also more likely to have lower back problems. We'll briefly go over the anatomy of your core muscles as well as those in your lower back. At the end of the section on arm anatomy, we'll take another look at the core, coming down from the shoulders.

> This is the highest area of the body where musculature connects directly from the legs. Your core is also connected to your arms and head, so it overlaps nearly all musculature systems in your body.

First the big one—what people call the abs. If you do a good crunch, or bend forward, you will feel three "stopping" points in your abdomen.

Just as we did with the other sections of your body, put one or both hands on your abs while you bend over and see if you can feel how this area moves. This is all one giant muscle, divided up into multiple sections. Officially, it's called the rectus abdominis, and no, that's not the name of a dinosaur from a *Jurassic Park* movie. This paired muscle (one on each side of your bellybutton) goes all the way past your sternum—that little nubbin in the middle of your chest—down to your groin. The reason it feels like a lot of small muscles (and why we call it a "six-pack" when you can see it on someone) is because there is a bunch of connective tissue between parts of the muscle, the fascia that I mentioned in the section on "interior" muscle. The "packs" are bundles of muscles, like a handful of straws. The connective tissue is the same stuff tendons and ligaments are made of, but they're not called that because neither end connects to bone.

So what? This band of muscle is the primary way we flex our spine forward. It connects your ribs to your pelvis and keeps most of your internal organs inside your body. It's also used in maintaining that semi-relaxed connection I spoke about above. When you stand up straight and expand upward, like you've been practicing this entire book (you have been practicing, haven't you?), this band of muscle engages from groin to rib cage. It's the largest area in your body that doesn't have a solid internal structure.

The only bones inside your lower torso are your vertebrae, which are only a few inches or centimeters around, and are in the back of your body. What's holding up all those juicy organs? This band of muscle. Along with your hips, this is one of the most important areas of your body to pay attention to in everyday action.

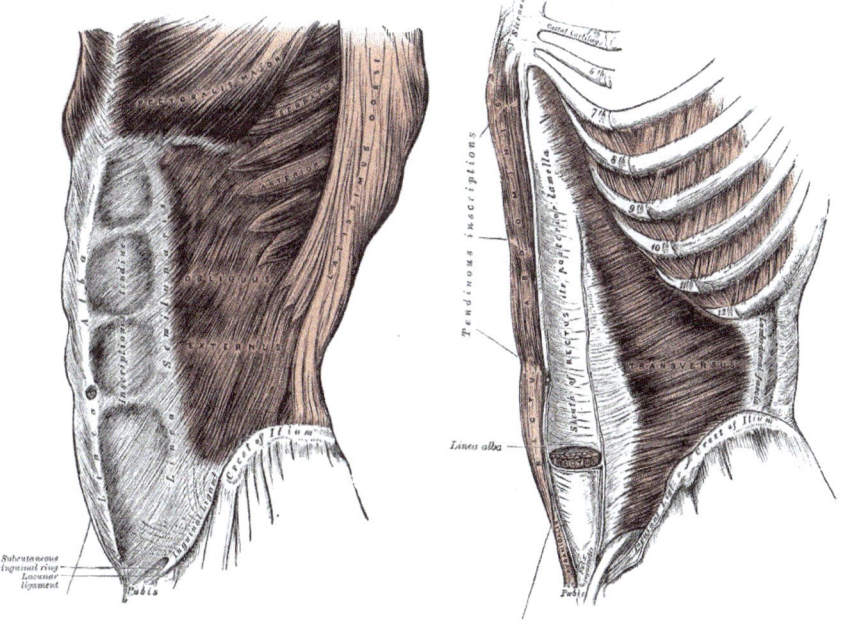

Figure 35: The muscles of the torso, notably showing the rectus abdominis and the bundles of musculature. The obliques are to the sides of the abs (Gray's Anatomy).

The abdominal oblique muscles are connected to the sides of the rectus abdominus, and basically do the same thing to the sides that the abs do in the front, though they don't have facia "packs." I'll talk about compressing the abs later on, and the function works the same way with the obliques. They're also very important in twisting motion. The obliques and the abs form a solid wall of muscle all the way across your front and sides.

Although your abs keep your rib cage from flopping forward over your hips, they don't actually connect your upper body with your lower body. There's only one muscle that does connect all the way from your spine to your leg bones, and that is the psoas (pronounced "soaz") major. This is an internal muscle, but it's the muscle that lets you pick your leg up while you're standing upright. Get in your good posture, then lift your knees up in front of you like you're marching. You're using your psoas major to do this work. If you march in place for a while, you'll start to feel a burn around the center of your leg. This is where the psoas connects.

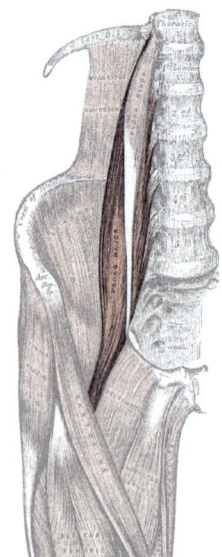

Figure 36: The psoas major, highlighted in the muscles of the groin and pelvis (Gray's Anatomy).

Let's move up to the back. As I said, the muscles in the back are just as important as those in your front. Your abs keep all that mushy stuff in your belly from falling out and they let you bend over. The psoas major lets you move your legs while you're standing or your upper body while you're lying down. But what resists that movement? How do you return from bending forward or lifting your legs up? Basically, how do you keep standing up straight (in good posture...) while you're moving around?

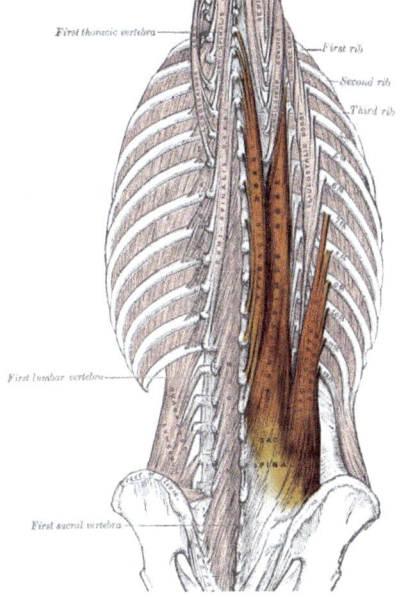

Figure 37: the erector spinae muscle group (Gray's Anatomy).

The main set of muscles responsible for this is called the erector spinae. This muscle set is made of three smaller sections that fan out from your spine to the middle of your back. You can feel this muscle set fairly easily if you put one hand on your spine, then feel the ropey lumps on either side of it. It helps to bend forward slightly. This is the largest of the three sections of the muscle set, and there's a matching pair, one on either side. Start from a standing posture and put your right-hand fingers on the right side of your spine and your left-hand fingers on the left side, near the small of your back. Now lean side to side, lean forward and backward, and twist your body between hips and shoulders. You should feel those ropey ridges relax and engage as you move. This band of muscle is what resists the motion of your abs in front. They don't have to be as large because they get a lot of extra support from your spine, and there are a lot of layers to these muscles. However, if you over develop your abs and don't work on this area, it can lead to back problems.

Another important muscle of your lower back is called the quadratus lumborum—no, that's not a spell to make a feather float. If you move your fingers out from your spine, past the erector spinae, and around your kidneys, there's another band of muscle. Technically, this is not a back muscle, but the most rearward of your abdominal muscles (which is why we're covering it here). It connects the top of your hip, your spine, and maybe even a rib or two (the actual connection varies from person to person). Now, you really don't want this muscle to take a lot of stress. If it is used to prop you up for long periods of time, it may get fatigued and lead to back pain. It is, in fact, the most common cause of back pain. Instead of relying on this muscle, it's better to develop your erector spinae to take the load, as that's what it's there for.

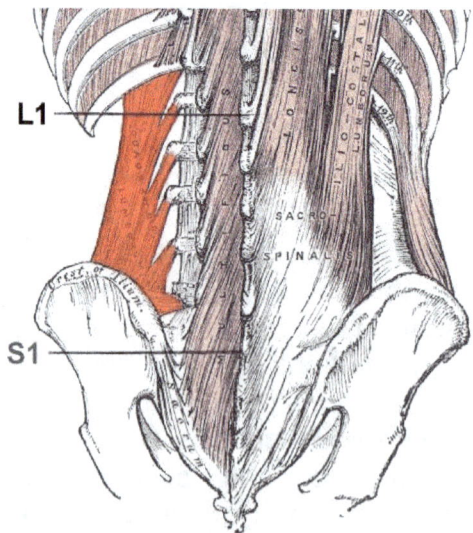

Figure 38: The quadratus lumborum muscle is highlighted (Gray's Anatomy).

Keep these abdominal muscles in mind while you move, with good posture. If you expand upward while you stand, like I've talked about, you should feel these muscles engage. Tucking your hips will keep the back muscles from compressing and losing effectiveness, and also lets your abs keep a good connection to your ribcage. We'll be coming back to these muscles from the other side after looking at the anatomy of the arms.

At this point, I've covered the lower body, and you have enough to understand the first section after the anatomy, concerning legs, leg movement, and walking. It's one of the main points of this book! So either skip ahead to that, or if your brain isn't too full with the muscles of the lower body, we'll move on to the upper body!

Anatomy of the Upper Body

In the previous section, I went through the connections from the feet up to the core. I'm going to do the same thing here, but this time I'll start from the fingertips, go up to the shoulders and neck, then down to the upper half of your torso. This won't include your center of mass like the anatomy of the legs does, and that actually tells a lot about the upper half of your body already: *it doesn't contain your center of mass.*

On the one hand, this is good because you can move the upper half of your body without shifting your feet or your stability. If you've ever stood on a ladder and kept your balance "back" while reaching with a hand so you don't fall off, you're compensating by only moving the part of your body without your center. This will be helpful for advanced manipulation in the body mechanics section. Your upper body is more dexterous because it can move independently of your connection to where you're standing (or sitting or lying down).

On the other hand (because you've probably got the two in your upper body!), this is bad because you can't affect your lower body with your upper body, unless you lean so far one way or the other your center starts to shift sideways (like the zombie arms exercise at the beginning of the book), or unless you connect your lower and upper body together through your core. This is a *really* important concept but requires knowledge of your full body. Stay tuned!

For now, let's go through the anatomy of the hands, arms, shoulders, neck, and chest.

Hands and Wrists

Hands are important. They're one of the major components that define us as human. That's a bold statement but, I believe, a true one. The level of fine manipulation we can achieve with our hands (the author says, as he touch-types on a keyboard while watching words appear on a screen), combined with the planning and pattern matching of our brains, makes us quite powerful and capable.

Let's mess with them.

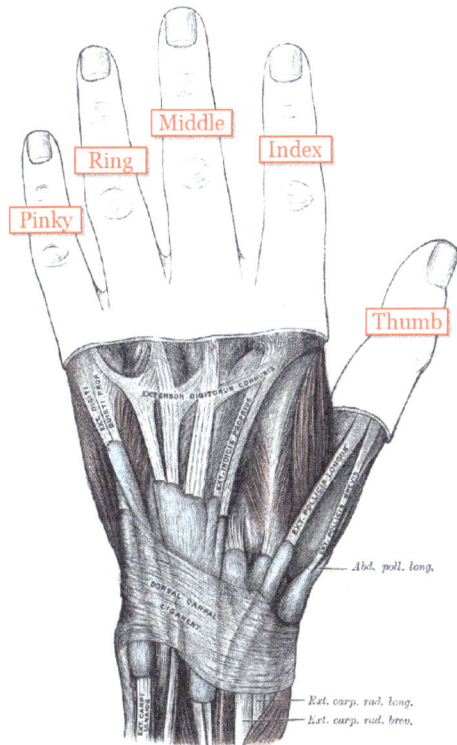

Figure 39: Overview of the hand, with fingers labelled as they are named in this text (*Gray's Anatomy*)

Try this: without looking, touch the fingertips of one hand to those of your other hand. I bet you could do this pretty easily, maybe adjusting a couple fingertips to make sure they lined up exactly. Did you have to look? Probably not. Try lifting each pair of fingertips away from each other and back together in turn. You'll likely notice more resistance with your middle and ring fingers than the others. Do you feel this resistance *in* your fingertips?

Probably not. Instead, it's about halfway down your forearm, isn't it? Keep that in mind.

Now with your fingertips touching, bring the heels of your hands to touch as well so your palms are completely touching. First, stretch your arms out in front of you, so your elbows are extended. Try to lift just your fingertips away from each other again. Probably about the same resistance for each, right?

Bring your hands, still together, back until your wrists touch your belly. Your arms should be in line with each other, elbows sticking out to each side, or maybe even bowed in a little, depending on your flexibility. Move your thumbs apart and back together. Now your pinky. Now your index finger (the one next to your thumb). Can you move your middle or ring finger at all? Why not?

If you can't, it's because you've just locked out the muscle that controls those fingers. If you can move your fingers, you've likely got some hyper-mobility in your joints.

Here's a fun fact: most of the muscles that move your fingers *are not in your hands*. The only muscles in your hands that aren't fascia (remember that?), or ligaments are the two meaty parts beneath your pinky and thumb on the palm side, and some very small muscles on the back side that loop around the base of your fingers and let you move them side to side.

Hyper-mobility is more common in women both from a nature side—estrogen tends to increase mobility of joints—and from a nurture side—women are more likely to participate in sports like dance, gymnastics, and skating, which increase flexibility.

Try putting one hand around your other arm, just forward of your elbow. Now move your free fingers and thumb. Are there any movements that *don't* move muscles in your forearm? About the only thing that doesn't (much) is to touch your thumb to your other fingers.

This brings us to another fun exercise: grasping. The human hand is almost hotwired to grasp. It's even a reflex in babies when their palm is touched up until about six months of age. We never really lose it. Place your relaxed hand over any light object and you'll start picking it up involuntarily.

Grasping uses those same forearm muscles. Lightly picking up an object barely uses them, as your hand naturally wants to grasp. When *gripping* or squeezing an object you can feel most of the muscles in your forearm contracting at once. You can get a very tight grip this way, but you're still not using all the muscles you could!

Try out a "crab claw" grip. Pinch the object using the muscles *in* your hand—the ones under your thumb and pinky. You might be able to get about the same strength as using your forearm muscles. Try this out with a full (unopened) plastic soda bottle, as it's easy to grasp and squeeze and will resist quite a bit of pressure. Squeeze with the forearm muscles. Then squeeze with the thumb and pinky. Now, it's a little harder to do, but try to squeeze with both sets of muscles at once. You can generate a very tight grip!

This grasping tendency can also be our downfall. We have an ingrained mindset to *keep gripping*. In martial arts, there are many ways to defend yourself when an opponent has grabbed your wrist or arm, by gripping them in turn, or manipulating their joints. The easiest way for the opponent to get out of these locks is to *stop grasping*, but almost no one thinks of that in the spur of the moment. Your hands want to grasp. Your fingers pull inward much more powerfully than they expand outward, which is why if you touch a live wire with your palm, you may not be able to let go, as the electricity will activate all those powerful gripping muscles and clamp on to the live surface! But if you accidentally touch with the back of your hand, you can pull away from the current.

While you've been following along, wiggling your fingers like you're trying to cast a spell, you probably moved your wrists as well. If your fingers are the ten dexterous points of precision for your hands, your wrists are the support system that can place your fingers in almost any position. The tops of your wrists are an extremely complex bunch of small bones, called the carpals. These are eight oddly shaped bones all stuck together between your wrist and about the base of your thumb. They don't take up much room at all, but each bone makes a tiny joint with the ones around it, as they're all connected by a bunch of ligaments that look like a spider had too much caffeine. Together, the carpals provide a flexible support structure for your fingers. They're not as strong or as load bearing as the small bones in your feet (the tarsals), but they're ready to support your daily manipulation needs.

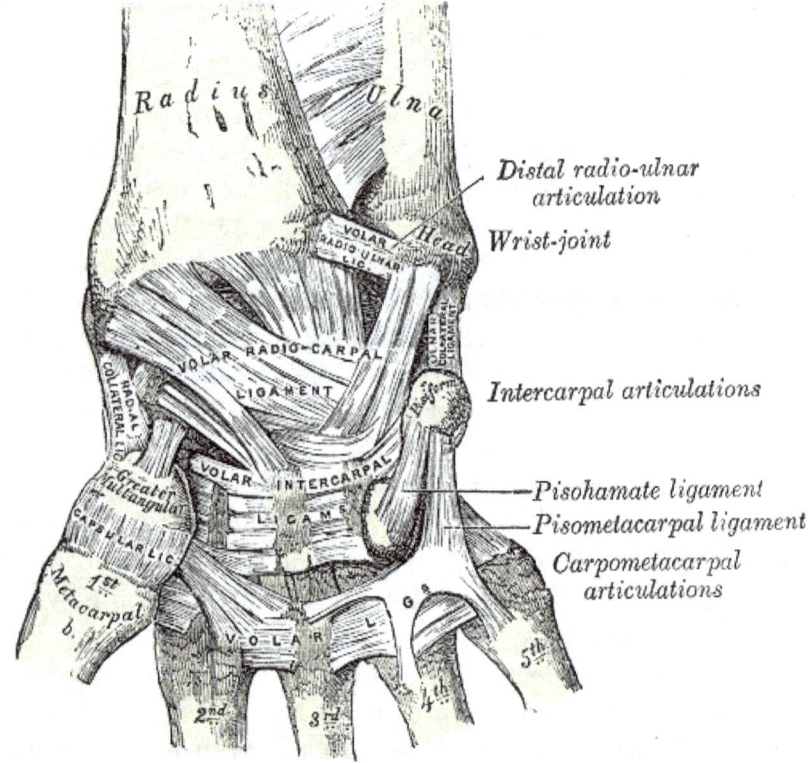

Figure 40: The spiderweb of carpal ligaments (*Gray's Anatomy*)

The bottom bones of your wrists are the ends of the two bones in your forearms, the radius and the ulna. But *in* the wrist? The actual connection between "arm" and "hand?" There are no bones. There are a *lot* of ligaments, tendons, and nerves. They all pass under a ligament connecting from one side of your carpals to the other, holding them in like a cable organizer for your computer, called the carpal tunnel. If this ligament gets inflamed for some reason, it might compress all those tendons and nerves, causing the pain known as carpal tunnel syndrome.

You can easily demonstrate that the wrist only has squishy parts in it rather than hard bone by this exercise. Take the thumb and index finger of one hand and place the thumb at the base of your hand directly under the bottom knuckle of your opposite thumb, on your opposite wrist, and your index finger on the other side of the wrist opposite from it. *Carefully* squeeze in a little. You'll feel there are not only no bones, but you can begin to separate your hand from the rest of your arm! Your hand might also flop forward as you squeeze in. If you squeeze too hard, you'll quickly feel pain in your wrist as you compress all those cables. The wrist is an excellent point of mobility in our body, only surpassed by the shoulder in the ways in can move. However, the lack of any solid structure in it also makes it a weak point during impact or falling, and why we do a lot of wrist manipulation in martial arts.

> Because of all the muscles and tendons in the arm, the wrist is one of the prime targets for manipulation in martial arts because lots of connections run through it and it's natural to grasp someone else's hands and arms with your hands.

To sum up, let's do one final exercise to show the mobility of the wrist. It's actually not as much as you would suspect, because it's supported by the movement of your arm and shoulder. Hold one forearm straight up in the air, so your wrist and hand are vertical and your fingers are pointing to the ceiling. Without moving any other part of your arm, let's go through the types of rotation. The first and easiest is to bend your hand forward and back, so your palm is down and then up. The second type of rotation is side to side. Your wrist can waggle a bit to the left and right, like Queen Elizabeth II waving.

And that's it! Your wrist only has two ways it can bend. The third method of rotation, twisting, is accomplished by the bones in your forearm, and that's what we're going to go over next.

The Forearm

Like your lower leg, your forearm has two parallel bones. Unlike the leg, both bones in your forearm are useful for hand manipulation. The radius is the one on the thumb side of your hand, and the ulna is the one on the pinky side. If we try the same exercise at the end of the last section, the radius and ulna are what create the third method of rotation for your hand, that of twisting. This ability is mostly found only in mammals, and those with hands that can grip and pull can make better use of it, for example, in climbing.

Your radius and ulna are the only two bones that cross and uncross in normal movement! Think of the ball and socket joints in your hips and shoulders. While those joints can go all the way around, the wrist only has so much rotation before you have to go back the other way. This is because when your palms are up, the radius goes from your thumb to the outside of your elbow. The ulna goes from the pinky to the inside of your elbow. Now turn your palms down. The bones still connect in the same place, which means the radius and ulna are crossing over each other.

In and around these two bones, surrounding them on a superficial and deep layer, are the muscles of the forearm, and there are a lot of them! There are a bunch of individual manipulators each connected to a fingertip, with names like "flexor digitorum superficialis," "extensor carpi ulnaris," and "pronator teres." Instead of memorizing what sounds like a wizard battle, let's feel it out.

Supination **Pronation**

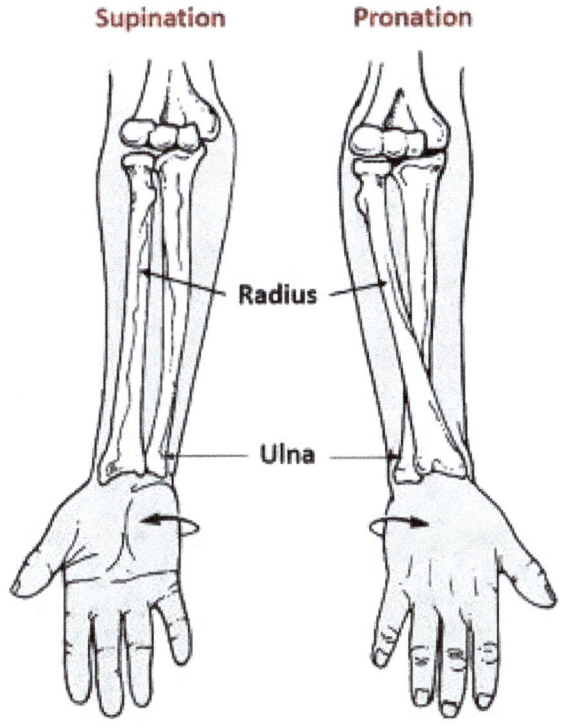

Radius

Ulna

Figure 41: The radius and ulna uncrossed (supination) and crossed (pronation). (Image from anatomyqa.com)

Put your arm out in front of you, palm up. One at a time, flex each finger forward, at the first or second knuckle. That's right, each finger has three knuckles (except for the thumb, which has two)! The first is the one closest to the base of your hand and the third is the one near the fingertip. While you do this, watch your wrist. You'll likely be able to see movement across your wrist as each finger moves. You can also see movement near your elbow as the muscle for that finger flexes. Try the same thing with your palm down. You might see large tendons in the back of your hand moving around like piano strings. Now, with palm up again, try to touch your fingertips to the inside of each finger's first knuckle (the top of your palm). You'll notice almost all the muscles around your forearm flexing at once.

A good stretching exercise for the forearms is simply to try out that radius/ulna crossover. Raise your hands in the air (like you just don't care) and torque those arm bones! Another nice release for all those forearm muscles supporting your wiggling digits is to give them a little massage. Encircle one wrist with your other thumb and index/middle finger—whichever feels better—with your thumb on the palm side of your other hand and pointing away from you. Grip as tight as you can, maybe using that crab claw grip, and slide your fingers down your arm. Your other fingers might curl in while you do this, because you're manually manipulating all those tendons. See Figure 42 for how this looks. Now reverse your grip so your gripping thumb is toward your elbow (pointing in to your body) and slide it down your arm again. You'll likely have more strength this way.

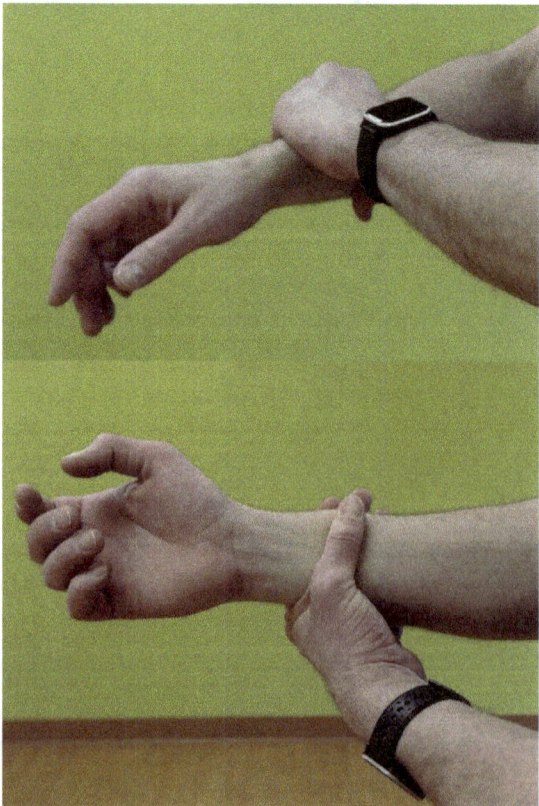

Figure 42: Massaging the forearm tendons.

One other warning about the forearm before we move on. Remember your radius is on your thumb side? The radius is also the bigger and studier of the two arm bones. The ulna is on the pinky side of your hand, but the way the bones are situated, the end of the radius supports the thumb, index, middle finger, and even a little bit of the ring finger (because the ring and middle finger share a tendon). The ulna only supports the pinky and some of the ring finger. This is why I tell my martial arts students that the pinky and ring finger knuckles are not "load bearing" when they punch.

Mammals that walk on all fours have their radius and ulna crossed when they do, for example a gorilla when knuckle-walking. When crossed, the radius and ulna are stronger than when they are side by side.

If you've ever practiced martial arts or boxing, you'll have heard to make contact in a punch with the first two knuckles only. That's because you can better transmit the force through the index and middle fingers down through your arm. If you don't punch things on a regular basis, be careful when putting weight on your fist, like supporting yourself on a table or pushing up from the floor. You can test this out and see. Make a fist (with your thumb on the *outside* of your fingers) and press into a hard surface, as in Figure 43. If you press against the first index and middle finger knuckles, it will feel stable. If you rock sideways so more pressure is on the ring and pinky fingers, you might be able to tell that it's easier to roll to the side or collapse your fist. Both of these can lead to wrist strains, so only use your load-bearing knuckles!

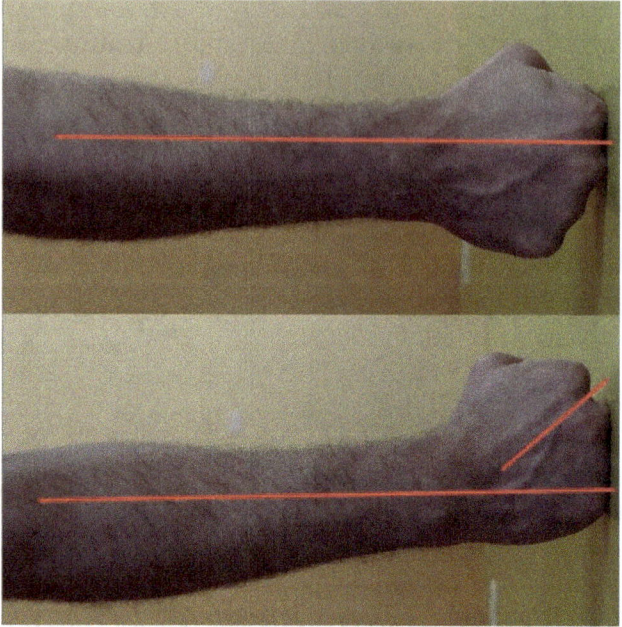

Figure 43: Aligning the "load-bearing" knuckles with the radius and ulna (top) and aligning the "non-load-bearing" knuckles with the radius and ulna (bottom).

Elbows

Ahh, the knees of the arms. Unlike the knees, elbows don't take as much constant stress, as you're not standing on them most of the time (unless you're an acrobat). Also, unlike the knees, the elbows don't have a separate piece of bone (the patella) that can be moved about and easily dislocated. But like the knees, elbows have a lot of interconnecting ligaments, that, if broken or torn, take a long time to heal, if ever. However, your twisting radius and ulna mean you don't have to keep your elbow positioned

> If your fibula and tibia (lower leg bones) were both connected to your femur (thigh bone) in the same way as your radius and ulna are both connected to the humerus (upper arm bone), you would be able to turn your foot 180 degrees like you can with your hands!

relative to your knuckles in any particular way, like you should keep your knees above your toes.

For the knees, I recommended squats to strengthen the small muscles around the joint and make them less susceptible to injury. What are squats for your arms? Pushups, of course. Either the wall pushups or chair pushups above are good to strengthen your elbows. If you want to build small muscle, the way to do it is high amounts of low weight, instead of low amounts of high weight.

Elbows are susceptible to falls, however! One of the easiest ways to dislocate your elbow is to fall forward and catch yourself with outstretched arms. The force goes through the heels of your hands, and travels up to the elbow, where it can push the joint apart. So if you feel yourself falling forward, bend your arms up toward your face! Hitting on the flat of your forearm dissipates the force rather than concentrating it at the elbow. You should also turn your head to one side so you don't smack your nose. Don't practice this now, there will be an entire section on falling!

Upper Arms

We're getting closer to the powerhouse of the upper body, but we're not quite there yet. Biceps look important and are a fairly large muscle in the upper body, but they aren't as powerful as you would expect. If you look at the thighs in contrast, which wrap around the femur and join far up into the pelvic area, the biceps only connect in relatively small areas to the elbow and forearm, and into the shoulder. If you think about it, the biceps are analogous to the hamstrings, the smaller muscles on the back of the leg (which is literally named the "biceps femoris"), rather than the quadriceps that gives most of the bulk to the front of your thighs. See Figure 44.

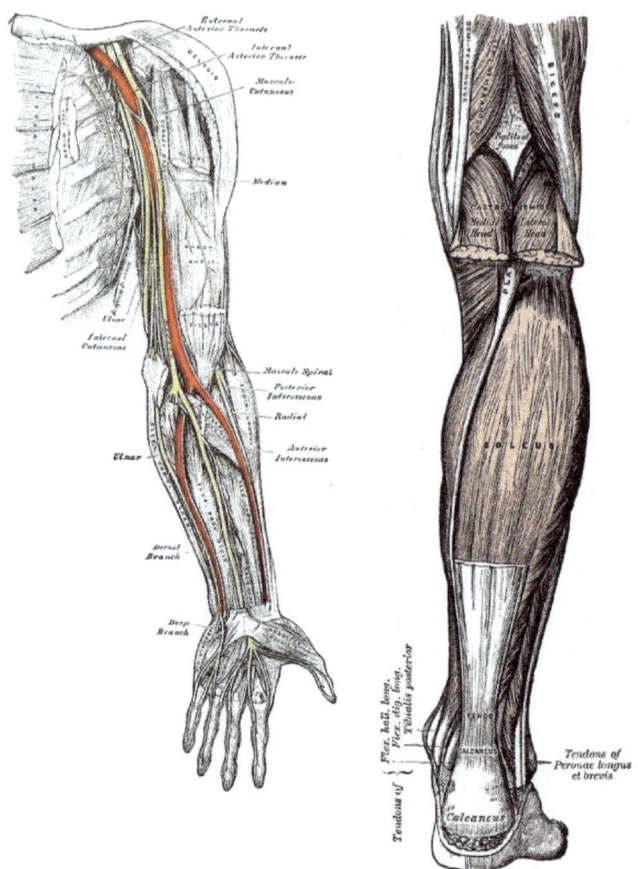

Figure 44: The muscles of the arm (left) vs. the muscles of the leg (right). Note the biceps is more equivalent to the hamstring muscles (*Gray's Anatomy*).

So why am I being so negative about the biceps? Mainly because popular culture puts a lot of emphasis on them rather than the other muscles that surround them. The triceps, on the underside of the arm, are more analogous to the quadriceps, and more solidly connected through the shoulder joint and into the elbow.

There's another big difference between the muscles of the upper arms and those of the upper legs. With the legs, the muscles are connected close to the center of your body. They can carry your weight, and the rest of your body sits atop them. They are integrated. They're in a straight line with your movement.

Your biceps and triceps, in contrast, are only connected into the shoulder joint. Force through them goes directly into your shoulders and causes stress there, rather than being dissipated into your torso. This is one reason shoulder and elbow stress issues are very common. I'll show you ways to mitigate this stress in everyday movement in the second half of this book!

Humans have adapted to be bipedal, which helped us create a civilization, but also has some other drawbacks. Think about how our limbs would be situated if we walked on all fours. Look at your cat or dog for comparison. On all fours, both the legs and the arms are putting force into the middle of your body, more or less in a straight line. In this case, your hands are pressing on the floor and the force is going up to your shoulders, then continuing up into your torso.

However, when you're standing up, force from actions with your hands is going up to your shoulders, then what? A lot of that force stops at the rotator cuff and shoulder cap.

That is, unless you know how to redirect the force and use your shoulder correctly... (dun dun duuuun!)

Shoulders

I went on about hips for a while in the anatomy of the legs. Well strap in. We've reached the hips of the upper body.

There are a ton of small and large muscles—near the surface and deep—that wrap around your pelvis and up into your torso from your legs. Just take a step with your hands on your hips and you can feel all those muscles moving. Your shoulders are very similar. Put a hand on your opposite shoulder and move that shoulder's elbow in a circle. Up past your biceps and triceps, there are a lot of overlapping muscles that tie your upper arms to your ribcage in the front, and the ribs and spine in the back. *This* is where most of your upper body power comes from, not your biceps or triceps, because it ties to the center of your body.

Remember your posture? I haven't been nagging you much about it for a while—sorry. While you've been feeling your shoulder, is it forward, or where it's supposed to be, above your rib cage? Shoulders go up, back, and down to reset them where they should be. Another way of doing this is by "lowering" your shoulder and back muscles.

Tying the motion of your arms to your center has to occur through manipulation of your abs. In the legs, moving around naturally carries your center with you. This is why it's easier to damage your shoulder muscles if you are very active, but not in proper posture with connection through your core.

The shoulder has a wider range of motion even than the hips do, largely because they don't need to support your body weight most of the time and thus can be used to position your hands in a wider variety of positions than your feet. Both joints are ball and socket, but the hips have a more complete "socket" around the ball end of your femur. The shoulder is resting against a shallower cup, like a golf ball on a tee. This gives it more mobility, but also means it's connected almost entirely by the muscle around it. This is why degradation in the hip is more likely to be a wearing of the ball and socket joint itself, whereas a shoulder injury is more likely to be a form of muscle or ligament tear. Both take a long time to heal, but a hip replacement can replace worn bone completely while a healed ligament in the shoulder might still be weak after it gets repaired. Neither is preferable if you can avoid them!

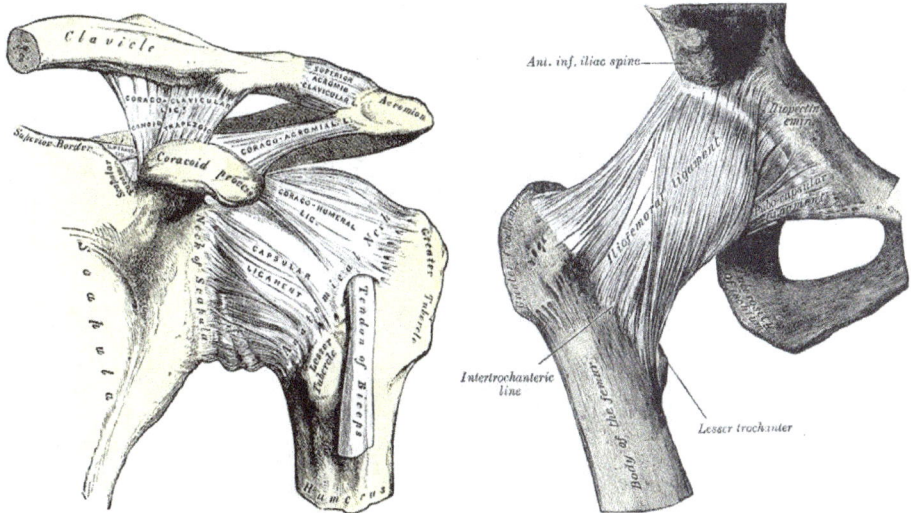

Figure 45: The shoulder joint (left) vs. the hip joint (right) (*Gray's Anatomy*).

Between your arm bones, your scapula (shoulder blade), and your ribs and spine, there are a bunch of muscles overlapping each other like a laminated pastry. On the inside are the supraspinatus and the infraspinatus, the teres major and teres minor, all connecting the top of your humerus to your shoulder blade. On the front side, the coracobrachialis muscle, which sounds sort of like it's supposed to be a seashell, connects from the shoulder joint to about the middle of the humerus, and helps you pull your arm in toward your body. You don't actually need to know all these names—they're just fun to say.

On top of them, the deltoid wraps around from the front of the shoulder to about halfway across the shoulder blade. This is the muscle you feel when you touch your shoulder.

Finally, we have the pectoralis and the latissimus dorsi muscles. You're likely familiar with the pectoralis, or "pecs," as they have as much of a fan club as the biceps. They are large, powerful muscles that help you pull and push, lift up and down. There's a major and a minor muscle as well, and the minor muscle acts as a stabilizer.

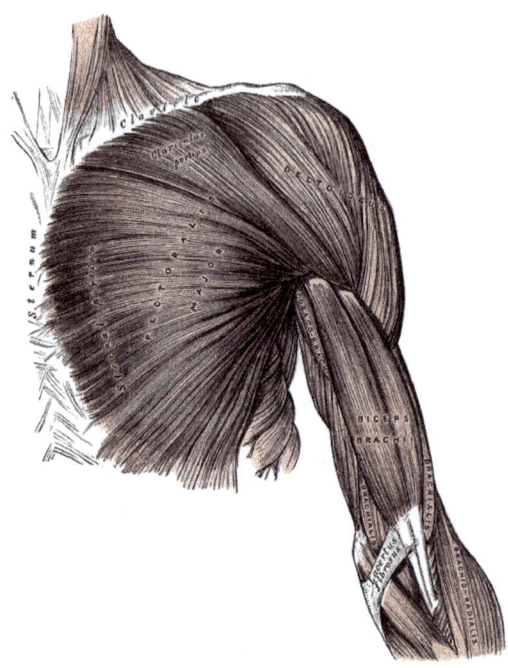

Figure 46: The shoulder muscles (*Gray's Anatomy*).

The issue with the admiration we heap on the pectoralis is that we often neglect the comparable muscles in the back that balance it, and working too much on the pecs when neck and back muscles are weak will make your shoulders and neck curve forward, leading to poor posture and back pain. Your back is supported by your spine, but on your front, the pecs don't have a strong connection to the abs, letting you slump forward.

In contrast, the latissimus (or "lats") is a huge sheet of flat muscle that connects the upper part of your humerus to nearly your entire spine below the shoulder blades, looking a bit like folded bat wings along your back. These assist in

The deltoid is comparable to the gluteus muscles around your hips. It even has three heads, or connection points, which line up somewhat with the gluteus minimus, medius, and maximus.

pulling things down from above, hanging and climbing, supporting yourself when leaning forward on an object. So remember to call out, "I'm Batman!" whenever you do a pullup. A tight or weak lat muscle can also lead to shoulder and back pain, especially paired with an overly strong pectoralis muscle.

Neck

We're going to take a quick detour up toward your head before going back down your spine, because this is the region where the trapezius sits. It connects on the other side of your shoulder blade ridge (that ridge of bone you can feel just over your shoulder) from all the little muscles in the shoulder blades that connect to the humerus. The trapezius then connects like a zipper all the way from your skull to your mid back and makes up that triangular ridge of muscle on the side of your neck. It's the one that feels so much better when someone kneads it to loosen it up.

In fact, let's take a quick aside to show a few good exercises to release some tension in your trapezius. A very easy one is to first put your shoulders in a good position (up, back, down), then put your arms straight out to the sides of your body, then bend your forearm upward, like you're trying to press your back and arms against a wall. Do this against a wall, if it helps. Then move your upper arms above and below your shoulders. It's surprising how much this loosens tense muscles! It might also make you yawn or stretch (or pandiculate!).

A second one—that takes greater hand strength—is to press your index and middle fingers directly into the opposite trapezius, right around the bony top of your shoulder. Then, keeping the same pressure, scoot

We're not fully covering the muscles of the head in this book, mainly because most of them are involved in moving your jaw, and because you generally don't want to interact with your surroundings (physically at least) with your head.

your fingers up your traps toward the middle of your neck. You'll likely feel a lump in the muscle that will "pop" as you move your fingers across it. Continue to do this until the lump and "pop" disappear (or until you feel better—sometimes it takes several sessions with some rest in between to get rid of all the lumps).

Finally, another good muscle release is to put the back surface of your thumb (the line between the two thumb knuckles) against the front of your opposite trapezius where it sits above your shoulder. There should be a little divot there, above your collar bone. Then hook the fingers of that hand over the trapezius and *squeeze* toward your thumb. Feel free to use the crab claw grip from above! You're activating the same muscle section that was "popping" in the above exercise. Experiment where you place your fingers and how much of the muscle you have between your fingers and thumb. I find it helps me to reach farther down my back with my fingers and "gather" muscle toward the thumb. Several strategic short squeezes in a row will knock out a lot of muscle tension. Reference the section on pain and discomfort above to help you realize how hard to squeeze and for how long.

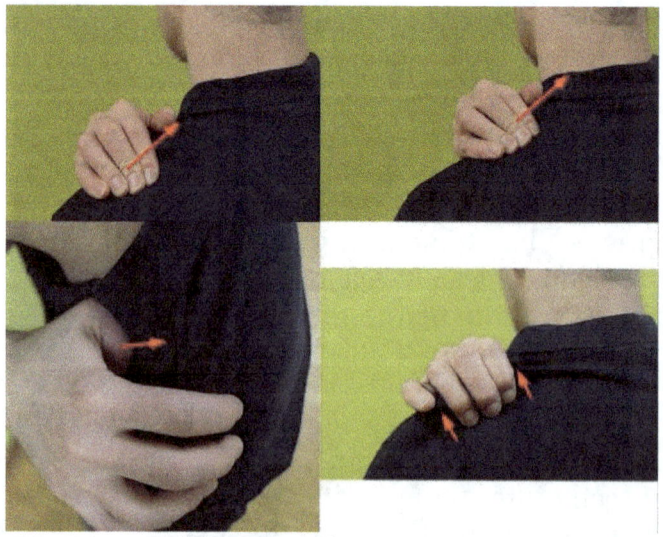

Figure 47: Top row: sliding across the trapezius. Bottom row: squeezing the trapezius. Note the thumb presses into the front of the trapezius to provide a stop to squeeze against.

Why do our trapezius muscles, in particular, get so tense? Part of it is that we tend to focus more on our front and less on our back. Another part is that a lot of us spend a lot of time looking slightly down at an angle when we really should be looking straight ahead. (I write this as I'm looking slightly downward at a laptop screen...) Remember way back at the beginning when I mentioned the head weighs as much as a bowling ball? So, when you tilt your head forward, off the centerline of your body, the first muscle it puts tension on is the trapezius. This "hunch" forward (of which I am just as guilty) puts constant tension on the traps and makes it bunch up into knots. This, in turn, leads to tension in the jaw and head and can cause all sorts of headaches and other mental malaise. So sit up straight when you use the computer!

In addition to this, a lot of us let our pectoral muscles—which are quite strong—bunch forward, further pulling on the trapezius. One thing you can do to combat this is to focus on the latissimus to help pull your shoulders down and back. Try to find the muscle that sits just under your armpit, toward your back. This is the top of the latissimus. Pulling it back and down a little will aid in standing up straight, combatting the pull of your pecs, and reducing stress on the traps. Try to keep this muscle in mind when you sit up. It will be hard to activate at first, but as you get used to it, it will become natural.

If you want to work your trapezius, here are a few exercises that can be done with or without weights. I'd suggest trying without weights to see if that releases some tension.

First, get in your good posture, then pull your shoulders toward the center of your spine, as above, hold it for two to three seconds, then release (Figure 48, left).

This is a good place to set a timer again and make sure you're sitting up straight, with your lats activated and head over your center!

Second, do the first part of resetting your shoulders. Lift them to your ears, hold a couple seconds, then release (Figure 48, middle).

Third, either standing or sitting in good posture, make fists and let your arms dangle. Then try to pull your fists up your sides, while bending your elbows. Hold for a couple seconds when you get as high as you can with your fists, then release (Figure 48, right).

Finally, do those wall pushups! Focus on your shoulders as you do, and let them bunch together around your spine.

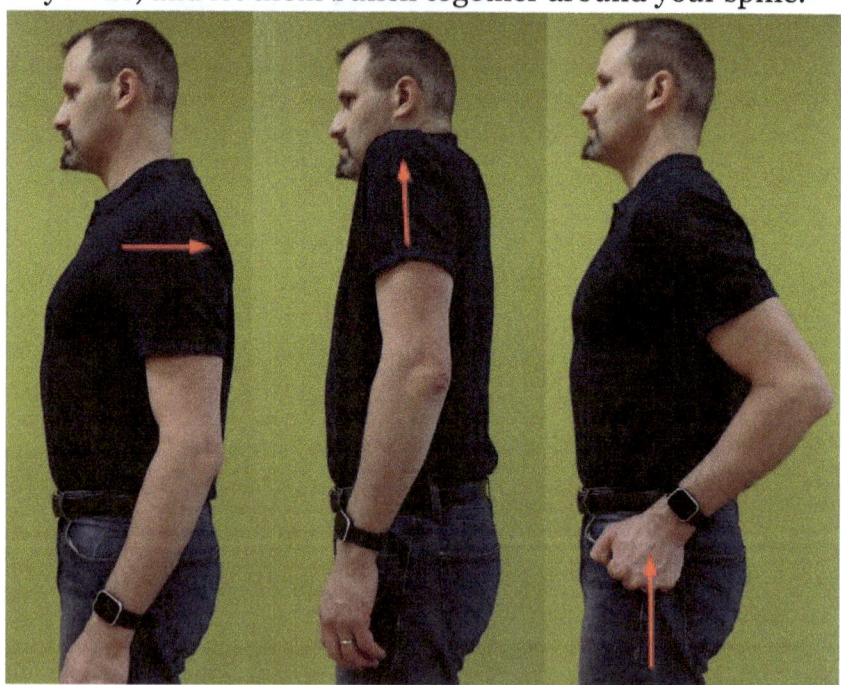

Figure 48: Left: pull the shoulders toward the center of the spine. Middle: pull the shoulders up. Right: pull arms up your sides.

Underneath the trapezius are the rhomboid muscles (major and minor) which help rotate and pull your shoulder blades backward. There are also the levator scapulae, which pretty much do what they say and lift the shoulder blades up. These muscles are certainly important, but in terms of injury and use, the rhomboids at least act as a sort of helper to the trapezius, so focusing on that larger muscle will also keep your rhomboids where they need to be.

Back

We covered the core in the section on leg anatomy, and we're getting to that same area again here, from the opposite direction. Your back is basically a wall of muscle (as is your front), but your back muscles are more closely connected to your spine, meaning they control how you move with much more mechanical ability. Try using just

The spine has five sections:
1) The cervical, which goes from your skull to your shoulders and has seven vertebrae
2) The thoracic, which goes from your shoulders to a little above your bellybutton and just below your ribs, is the most mobile part of your spine, and has twelve vertebrae
3) The lumbar, which stops around the top of your hips and has five vertebrae
4) The sacral and coccyx (sections 4 and 5), which are fused together and provide stability into your pelvis

your abs to turn your shoulders. Now try the same thing starting from your lumbar spine. It should be a lot easier.

At the center of all the back muscles is your spine. Not only is it a hub for transmitting electrical signals across your body, it's also the pillar around which your posture is situated. It's a bit of an evolutionary risk for us humans to stand up all the time rather than supporting our spine on all fours like most animals. It leads to a lot of back problems, but it also gives us superb tradeoffs in leaving both hands free to manipulate and carry.

The trapezius covers the cervical area of the spine, with the lower part covering the top half of the thoracic. The latissimus covers the thoracic area and reaches down into the lumbar area.

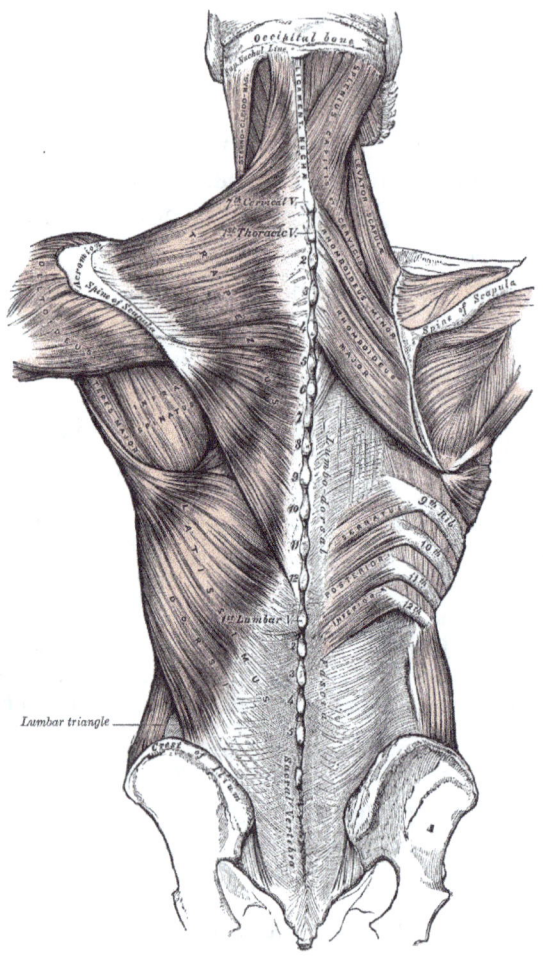

Figure 49: Muscles of the back. There are a lot (*Gray's Anatomy*).

The latissimus and trapezius (lats and traps) are the largest muscles and closest to the surface of the back, however, like the layers of tread in a tire, there are two deeper layers of muscle in the back. Learning a little about moving these, along with the surface muscles, will give you impressive control of your spine and overall movement. That's what you're here for, aren't you?

First off, there are the serratus posterior superior and inferior muscles. These two lie under the rhomboids and the latissimus and help with breathing and moving your ribs around. These muscles are not quite as important for overall movement, so I'm going to gloss over them.

Why are we putting so much attention into twisting your back? Because this is the primary connection between your upper and lower limbs. Controlling how your arms and legs interact with *each other* is important!

However, at the deepest level, there are some very powerful strings of muscle that run all the way up your back. These muscles develop all the way from the embryo stage, close to when the spine itself grows, and are very important for stability and balance. We covered the erector spinae above, but there are a lot of them, sounding something like a bestiary of mythical monsters:

The iliocostalis, longissimus, spinalis, semispinalis, multifidus, rotatores, interspinales, intertranversarii, and the levatores costarum. Reference Figures 37 and 38 in the section on the core for more detail.

These muscles are all so deep in your back that trying to isolate a single one is close to impossible. Instead, I'm going to ask to feel some things, and see if you can make your spine move around.

Let's start from the top. Find a comfortable seat and sit up straight with good posture (head up, shoulders back). If you can sit cross-legged with some lower back support, this will open up your lower lumbar area and make it easier to feel the effects there. If not, sitting with legs down is fine as well.

First, your head. Press up with your head, as if you're trying to reach the ceiling with it. The muscles along your spine are lengthening, stretching you out. It's a good way to decompress, and it helps you sit up straight. Just remember to keep your hips tucked in at the same time! From here, if you turn only your head (slowly) left and right, you should be able to feel the pull of the two muscle sets between your neck and shoulders (called the splenius capitis and splenius cervicis, if you care). There will be a little pressure right at the base of your skull. Now bring your head back to center and turn your whole upper body from a place on your spine directly behind the bottom of your ribcage. It's a much different feeling, and should turn your shoulder and head at the same time. This is using those deep muscles (and probably a little of your latissimus).

Let's go farther down. Still keep your good posture, with your head reaching toward the ceiling. This time, focus right above your hips, at the bottom of your lumbar area. Try to rotate your whole upper body from right above your hips. This is harder than rotating from your rib cage, simply because you're moving more mass. It's a bit like imagining each hip is pushing that side's shoulder forward. This action is using the multifidus muscle, one of the most powerful in the lumbar region, and not one we pay much attention to!

One last exercise in this area, but this one can be used to help lower back pain! Good posture again and pay attention to your lumbar area (lower back). Remember, there are five vertebrae here. Try to "lift up" above each vertebrae and "pull down" below it. This is more of a feeling than an exact science. Remember that all these muscles are densely packed around your spine. Fix a picture in your mind of your spine and vertebrae (See Figure 50). It doesn't really matter if it's accurate. What you're doing is focusing your attention on this area, and when you do that, you can start to directly affect the muscles there. You do technically have control over almost every muscle in your body, but most of the time you let your body do what it's accustomed to. This is purposefully changing how you move.

I find it easier to start this exercise at the very base of the spine, where the lowest mobile vertebrae connects to the sacrum (that hard section at the base of your spine). Again, fixing a picture in your mind, push your sacrum *down* and pull the rest of your spine *up*. Then move a little farther up your spinal column and repeat. Eventually, you can make this feel like a rolling wave up your lower spine, and is a great way to decompress that area. I find it helps to have a solid lumbar pillow to press back against as you try this so it doesn't distort the curve of your lower spine. You can also experiment with pulling right and left as a sort of "wiggle" to add to the movement. I've felt vertebrae pop back into alignment when doing this exercise. Just a caution not to overdo it, especially if you haven't tried moving your muscles like this before, or already have chronic back pain. Just like everything else, start small and work up to fully operating your body.

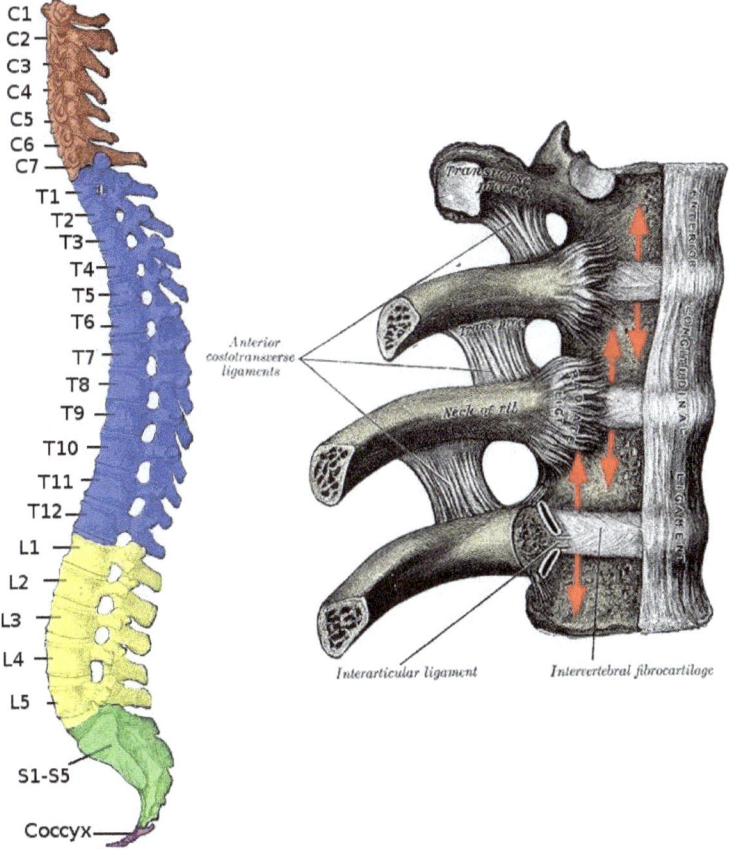

Figure 50: The five sections of the spine, along with a closeup of how to visualize "separating" vertebrae. (Attr: Henry Vandyke Carter, Public domain, via Wikimedia Commons)

This is the end of the anatomy section, but I'm going to reference things in here quite a bit in back half of the book, so feel free to reference something if you don't remember. I have a good bit more to say about your core, as well, but you're going to need some practice before being able to feel what I'm talking about. It's a more complex motion. For now, let's learn how to walk and lift!

How to Walk!

We've gotten this far and I'm just now getting to how to walk? Yes. That's right. The reason it's taken so long is that I wanted you to be thinking about all the interconnected parts of your body, so you have the groundwork when I cover a complete and coordinated action, like walking. Walking does, in fact, use almost everything I've talked about so far. Even the parts you think it doesn't. *Especially* those parts.

Yes, you might think walking is easy, since you've been doing it nearly your entire life. This is false. Often while in public, I watch people walk, mostly paying attention to their feet. If you do this, you'll see there are many different methods people use to walk. Some are more efficient than others.

If you get shoulder or neck pain after walking for a long time, you probably aren't standing up straight. Go back and practice. If you are getting lower back pain, you likely aren't connected between your hips and your shoulders. Really work on tucking your hips in and extending your upper half so you connect your hips and shoulders. Remember the exercise with your head connected by a string to the ceiling (or connected to some sort of strange skyhook if you're outside). When you don't walk as efficiently as you could, your muscles get more tired than they need to be. The section about posture at the beginning of this book is only the first step (ha). You have to practice a lot to make it innate. I've been doing this for years and I still lose my posture.

If you've gotten to this point and you haven't done those exercises I described, **stop, go back, read them again, and try them out.** I promise that understanding—and by extension, practicing—them will make a big difference to reading the rest of this book. That is, after all, the reason you're reading it, isn't it? Otherwise, you're just nodding along with the cool things I'm saying, but not paying attention to them.

Seriously, go back to that very first section, and practice with the timer like I said. You'll need some sense of your muscles so you understand the connection all the way from your feet to your core. Get at least a week of stretching in to start feeling some of the benefits. Relax. Set a timer along with your posture so you remember not to tense up. The worst culprits are usually shoulders and neck. Don't let your shoulders rise up into your ears.

Go on. The book will still be here when you come back.

...

Have you spent a while feeling things out? Can you recognize when you're losing your posture? Have you started stretching? If so, you may be ready to learn how to walk. Cue angelic music.

The Mechanics of Walking

If you've done everything above (actually done it. I've got my eye on you...), then let's go through what happens when you walk. I know you've been doing this unsupervised—with no expert in sight—for many years. Just pretend you're learning it for the first time.

Unsurprisingly, the first thing to do when trying to walk is to have good posture. You should be used to this by now and can hopefully even keep your good posture without me telling you to. But of course, I'm going to go over it again. Head up, shoulders back, hips tucked, knees slightly flexed. Pretend you have a string tying the very top of your head to the ceiling, always in tension. Extend through your core so your hips are connected to your shoulders. When you stand, reach upward, away from the ground. Think about expanding your body, rather than compacting it into a smaller space. In other words, what your mother always told you: don't hunch.

Got all that? Now we are going to walk and chew bubblegum—except I'm all out of bubblegum, so we're going to walk and hold posture.

I want you to feel the differences between efficient and inefficient movement. So, first we're going to do it the bad way. Shake everything out. Remember how you used to stand (before I came along and showered you with amazing advice).

As much as it pains me, I want you to go back to your normal posture, or even accentuate bad posture. Slump, hunch forward, have your shoulders up, head forward, hips untucked, belly out, whatever. Go for a little walk, making sure to walk forward for at least twenty feet. Try to walk backward as well and see what happens when you turn in a circle or even try to step sideways. Don't pay attention to how your feet move. We'll get to that in a minute. You might feel like you're not really getting anywhere when you walk. In fact, I hope this feels gross and awful and you never want to do it again. Because now we are going to fix it.

No pressure. Stand in good posture. Head, shoulders, hips, knees, connection, extension.

> Even if you don't feel anything, don't worry. The next exercise should make the difference clearer.

I want you to go for a little walk. Don't pay attention to your feet yet. Just worry about keeping that posture and connection intact. Don't even take this book with you because I don't want you to be looking down (but read the rest of this paragraph and the next first so you know what you're doing). Look straight forward when you walk so you don't tilt your head up or down and accidentally ruin your posture.

Here's what I want you to do: walk about twenty feet forward, then stop and walk backward. One of the things I always find hardest is keeping your hips tucked while you're walking. Make sure they don't sag and lose connection with your core and shoulders. Next, turn in a complete circle with your head still upright in good posture (remember that posture). Finally try stepping sideways. Go do this, then come back and read the next section.

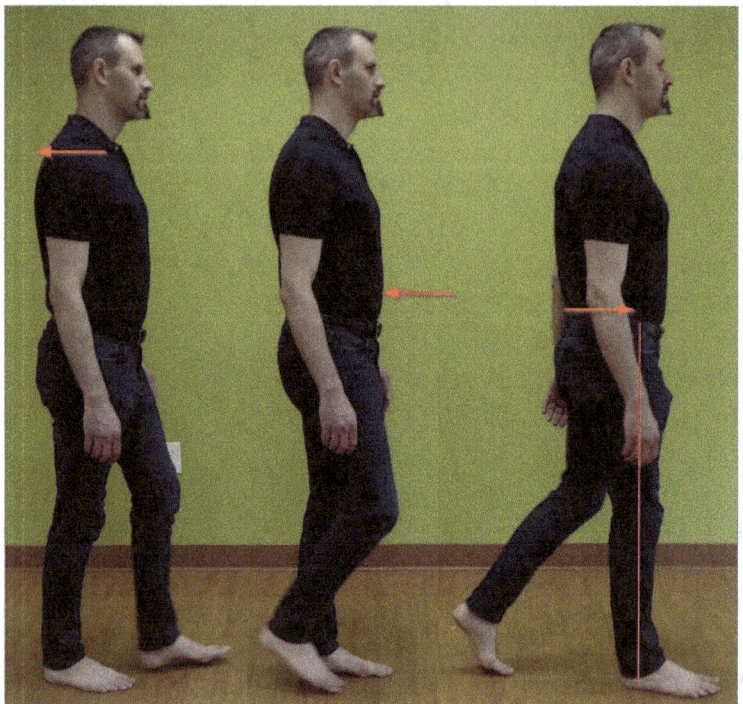

Figure 51: Walking with correct posture. Note the shoulders are back, the abs are connected to the hips and shoulders, and the center moves forward while walking, above the newly planted foot.

How did you do? Did it feel different than the first time? If you've gone from having no connection to full connection, walking should feel a lot "lighter," more fluid, and more coordinated than what you did before. You may feel like you're walking slower, yet covering the same distance you used to. Why? Because you've aligned your center of mass underneath you, rather than in front of you. You've also created a light connection all the way from your feet to your shoulders. You're not fully tense, but you're not completely relaxed either. Especially when moving backward, sideways, or turning, you should feel it's much easier to adjust your direction because your center of mass is closer to where all the action is happening: your hips.

Let's go back to the description of finding the center of mass for a minute. You don't need to actually hang yourself up on a wall, but if you imagine yourself in a flat plane (standing straight, with good posture) rather than in a curve (slumped forward), you can visualize that the center of your mass will be on the flat plane you make by standing up, rather than out in space in the middle of the curve from your hips to your head. Notice the straight line in Figure 52. It starts in the same place on the foot, but goes through the middle of the hip and the middle of the ear on the picture with good posture, and through neither on the one with poor posture.

On the other hand, if visualizing stuff like this makes your head hurt, don't worry about it. Just remember, if your body is in a straight line rather than a curve, then it's easier to move.

We're going to get into more complex analysis from here on out, and I want to make sure you have the fundamentals down—the fundamentals being everything up to this point. And you thought walking was easy.

Try to combine walking with the timer you use for posture and relaxation. You want to do all three at the same time (you can do all three at once, right?) so you don't put any extra effort into walking. Efficiency comes from the least energy input for the maximum work output. You can walk longer, farther, and with less stress on your body by using less energy to do it.

Remember how I said everything is about your hips? Does that make more sense now? While getting your upper body posture correct is challenging, I find being aware of how your hips move is even harder and takes a lot longer to master.

Try to walk and hold posture. You're still all out of bubblegum. Go practice again and try to remember all the things I've talked about. Good posture, hip to shoulder connection, relaxation, keeping your center in line, least effort. Try to keep all of this in mind. Okay, go on and take a walk.

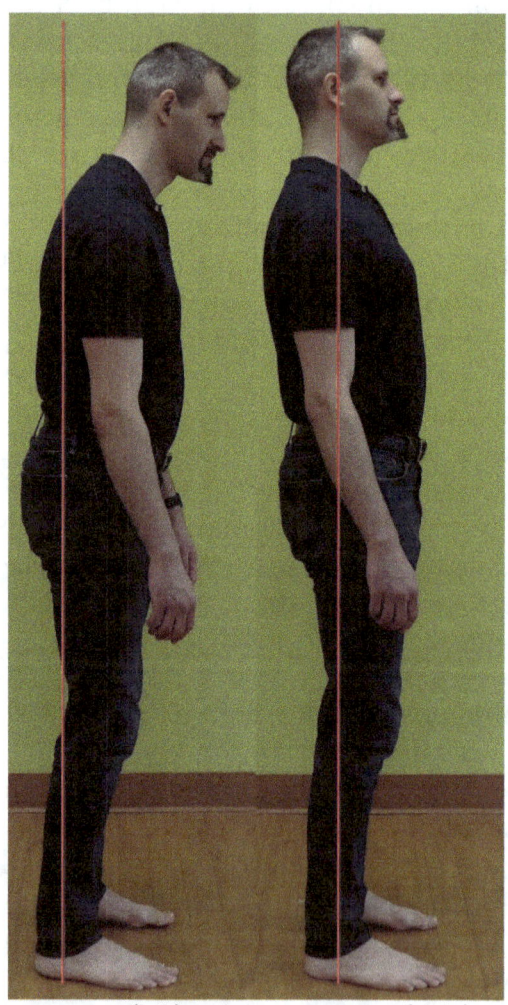

Figure 52: Poor posture (left) and correct posture (right). Notice the center of mass (red line) goes through the heel, waist, and ear when in correct posture.

I'll wait here.

...

Don't worry, I'm still waiting.

...

Have you practiced your walking? If you've done this over a period of several days, then are you starting to make this a habit? Does your walking gait feel better? Can you go faster with little effort? You might find yourself passing people who are suddenly walking so slowly. If you *have* practiced, everything I've talked about should start to become second nature. I hope it has, because we're really going into the deep end now. Deep breath.

> Time to practice again. I don't mind if you put the book down at this point and simply work on absorbing this concept for a week or so. You can just...uh...walk away from it.

How Your Feet Move When Walking

I told you to ignore your feet in the last part for a reason. I have a whole section about it here, so let's talk about your feet. Now you're aware of the basics (lots of them!) of walking, we're going to break down some tangential parts and see how they affect the whole.

This part will be easier to do without shoes, but if you have them on, that's fine. Just make sure you pay attention to what the different parts of your feet are doing in your shoes. Whenever you get a chance, try the same exercises with bare feet.

How do your feet contact the ground when you walk? Do you go heel-toe, heel-toe? Humans have walked in different manners throughout history, but for right now, in a society where we use shoes that have good support and are long-lasting, I'm going to say that heel-toe is the best method for how your feet should contact the ground during a regular walking gait. Let's look at some of the other methods in comparison. A lot of the inefficiencies I see with how people walk come from putting your feet to the floor in a different sequence.

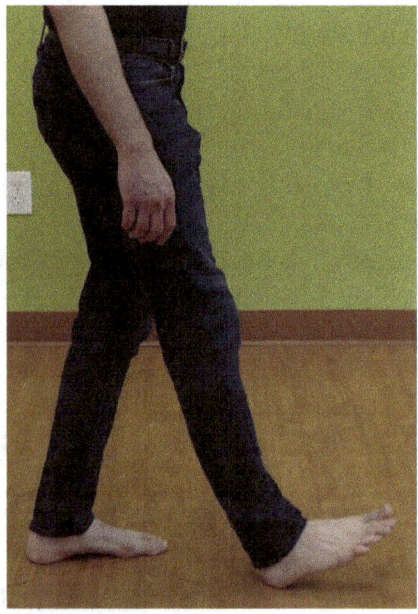

Figure 53: Walking heel-toe.

Some put their full foot on the floor at one time, stomping around with every step. It's more common with people who are hunched forward. If you use good posture, this is actually pretty hard to do because placing the full length of your foot on the ground at one time means your center of mass needs to be over the center of your foot. If you have good posture, your center of mass is going to be nearer your heel. Walking with the full flat of your foot also reduces the amount of flex through your foot, which can be bad for your tendons and for your knees. Wearing shoes that don't bend or are worn out might make this issue worse. If you're not able to roll your foot from heel to toe when touching the floor because it's encased in a heavy, unyielding material, you're more likely to walk flat-footed.

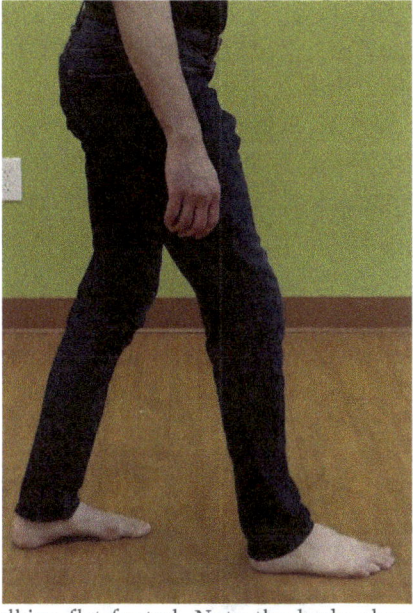

Figure 54: Walking flat-footed. Note the body above the waist is bent forward more.

Others walk on their toes, which, while good for some types of running (and for being sneaky), is not as beneficial for walking. When walking like this, your Achilles tendon (remember, that's the big springy thing that connects your heel to your leg) gets very tight. You can even strain it by walking on your toes for long periods of time. On the other hand (foot?), walking on your toes for short periods of time can work on your balance and muscle tension. But just like

If you walk in heels, the Achilles tendon is shortened and relaxed, passively. Standing on tiptoes is done by contracting the tendon, so it's active. Thus, an Achilles tendon strain can be treated using cowboy boots, which allows the tendon to relax.

lifting weights, you don't want to do it all the time. If you've walked in high heels for hours or even minutes, you probably understand this.

Another point worth mentioning is that walking toe-heel, or even only on the toes, is common among neurodivergent people. As I've said above, there's good reason to work on changing this walking method if you do it. Aside from issues with the Achilles tendon tightening, you can see in the comparison below how it affects your balance and efficiency (see Figure 55).

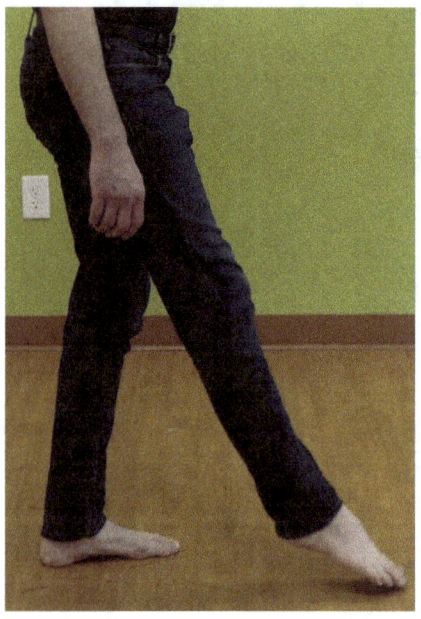

Figure 55: Walking toe-heel. Note the center is more over the back foot.

The method of walking that's hardest to diagnose, and the one I find most insidious in terms of ruining your posture and walking gait, is "bouncing" while you walk. This method is hard to see. If you look at someone's feet while they walk, your eye naturally goes to the foot that's taking a step, rather than the one that's still on the ground. Your eyes are attracted to movement. If you force yourself to focus on the foot that stays on the floor, you may see the heel pop up before the person finishes the next step. This little "pop" while walking causes all manner of inefficiencies and breaks your connection with the ground, and with your posture.

Remember how I said efficiency means using the least energy to do the most work? If you pop or bounce while you walk, you're doing more work in order to get the same job done. That "pop" in your stationary foot means even if you have good posture, you're rocking your whole body forward over the front of your foot. Can you imagine where your center of mass goes as you do this? To maintain posture, if you're even able to, you would have to pull your entire weight back from your toes to your heel. While it's a shift of maybe six or seven inches, you're shifting your entire mass backward while your intention is to walk forward. You're putting energy into going in the opposite direction to the one you want to. Most people who walk this way don't even try to correct their posture, as most of them aren't aware they're doing this.

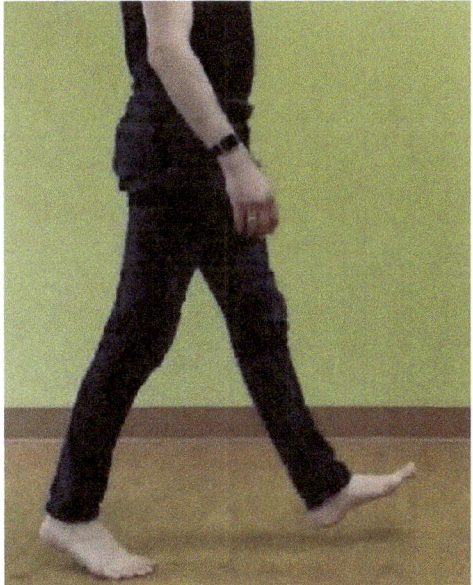

Figure 56: Walking with a bounce or "pop." Note the center is disconnected from the ground.

Instead, the person leans forward while walking and is forced to use their back muscles to compensate for their head being over their toes rather than over their heels. If they already have a slump forward in their neck and shoulders, this only exacerbates the problem. I guess what I'm saying, in short, is: don't walk this way.

Now that I've gone through (or ranted about) some of the ways you shouldn't walk, let's try heel to toe walking. This is going to feel silly, like something you already know how to do, but stay with me. Even if you don't think you need to do this, try it out, just in case.

Start, as always, with good posture. Remember to tuck those hips. Now, *without moving your upper body, or leaning or moving forward at all*, put one foot out in front of you, heel pointing down to the floor and toes raised at about a 30-degree angle from the floor. Let your heel settle to the floor. You'll probably have to shift your balance sideways over your support leg just a little to keep from leaning. Also, since you haven't moved your center of mass forward, you may also feel tension in your rear leg. That's because we've only done half of what you need to do to take a step.

Let's add the second part. Go back to where you were, standing up straight with your feet together. Now when you put the foot out in front of you, move your hips over your rear foot until they are over your toes instead of your heel. This will look a lot like Figure 53. You are shifting your balance forward while you do this, as well as shifting sideways to balance as you did in the first example. In order to keep your balance and keep from falling, your heel will land on the ground. Do you feel the difference between moving your center and not moving your center?

Tl;dr:
Step 1: put your foot out without shifting your hips forward.
Step 2: Do the same thing, but shift your hips forward this time. You'll feel your weight settle differently.

This is why I talked about your hips and your center of mass so much at the beginning of the book. They are central (quite literally) to how you walk.

Let's take a different example, just to show you why I like heel-toe better than the other methods of foot movement. Do what you did the first time— stand up straight and reach one foot out, but this time instead of pointing your heel at the floor, point your toes at the floor. When you touch the floor with your toes, you'll notice there isn't as much pressure on the rear leg as there is when you touch with your heel. You also don't really have to move your center. This is why it's good for sneaking around (see the explanation in the box). You don't have to commit your center to the movement, and you can test the ground where you're going to take a step.

> Watch how far you put your foot out when taking a step. You don't need to take a giant step, but your stride should be just long enough so you do have to move your center forward while stepping. If you don't move your center, you can step very quietly, but won't get anywhere fast.

But for these purposes, if you walk toe-heel, toe-heel instead of the other way around, you put less pressure on the back leg and you don't move your center forward. You *can* move your center forward if you walk this way, though you're less likely to, naturally. So why do I not prefer this method of walking? Because you *want* some tension between your body parts. Think of the stretching exercises, especially the isometrics. Creating a little tension can show you the most efficient line of motion. The muscles that get tense indicate you're at the extent of your available movement and must now move other parts of your body to continue.

When you have pressure that makes you move your hips forward, you will innately start to shift them forward earlier in the step. Why is this necessary? Because when you move parts of your body in coordination, rather than one after the other, it's more efficient.

Let's try one more example to show you why I prefer heel-toe. I'm going to make you imitate the dreaded heel popping. Oh no! Those who walk this way, I'm glaring at you (you can't see it, but I am).

By now, you should know to start with good posture. Like we did in the first example, stick one foot out, heel pointing toward the floor, move your hips in, and let your heel land. So far, so good. Here's that insidious balance shift that comes along with popping. I want you to *keep* shifting your balance over your front foot and lift up your rear heel up at the same time. You're standing on the toes of your rear foot and the heel of your front foot, and as you roll

> The total energy to move two body parts together is less than moving them one at a time. This is a more difficult concept to grasp, so if you don't fully get it, don't worry yet. We're still just focusing on your feet.

to put your front foot flat on the ground, your center must shift farther than normal and end up over your front toes. See Figure 56 for reference. So even before you finish your step, your center is too far forward. When you bring your back leg through, your center of mass is over the toes of your stationary foot rather than over the heel. It's as if you're continuously falling forward. The only way to stop this is to bring your entire body backward as I described above, which takes more energy than necessary.

> Aside from inefficiency, there's one other reason I despise "pop" walking. One key word: fall. You should always be in control of where your body is moving, but while walking with a "pop" you're falling forward because you're not in control of your center.

To make this even worse, most people don't have good posture (like you do, after all that practice!). So, try the same example as above, but this time, lean your shoulders and head forward (like I told you not to) as you step. If you pop your rear heel up as you are walking, and your shoulders and head are forward, your balance will be even farther forward, and you cannot help but fall onto your new foot, often sending a shock through your front leg. This is bad for your Achilles tendon and your knees, as well as being inefficient. This method of walking encourages you to have bad posture in order to fall into your next step. You are never completely in control of your motion, and you're making walking a high-impact sport.

Hopefully these examples explain why I like walking heel-toe. If not, read through the section above again. Go very slowly and feel out what I'm describing. Look at the pictures and compare them to what you're doing. There are a lot of subtle complexities, and it may well take a few read-throughs and trying it out for yourself to understand.

Now, try the heel-to-toe method. Good posture, from head to shoulders to hips and knees. Feel where your center of mass is, and as you take a step, move your center of mass *with* your front foot moving rather than before or after it moves. As soon as you pick up your front foot, your hips should also start forward.

Congratulations! You just took your first step (ha ha!) toward walking efficiently!

Time for a pop quiz! I did say there would be a test later. Which way do you walk? If you don't naturally walk heel-toe, try to figure out why. Are you not moving your hips forward when you walk? Are you leaning forward? Are you popping and falling forward? Feel how your thighs, glutes, and core move. Take twenty or thirty minutes to go over these different walking methods and try to understand how they do and do not work. You may have corrected some of your worst habits already if you've been practicing with correct posture. At least that's my hope.

Using Both Legs to Walk

Before moving on to this section, take some time to process the sections above. There's a lot crammed in there. Even if you set this book down for a week or two and try everything out, that's fine. Especially if you're making changes to your stance and the way you walk at the same time—for example, getting rid of the habit of popping while you walk—it can take a while before your body gets used to it. Don't worry. The book will still be here.

Remember what I said at the very beginning: from posture, to body connection from your feet to your head, to the way you place your feet when you walk, I've covered some major adjustments to how you operate your body. Once all those changes start to gel, *then* it's time to move on to the rest of this book. From here on, we are going to refine ever smaller pieces of how you move to get the maximum efficiency.

What helps the most in learning to do something new or different with your body is to *feel* what your body is doing as you move. You won't understand how to truly operate your collection of bones, muscles, and organs unless you know exactly what each muscle is doing. You don't have to know the fancy names or anything, as long as you pay attention to how you move. As I practice martial arts and body kinematics, even when I'm just walking around, I sometimes go down to the level of tensing and contracting one muscle at a time to figure out what it does and how it affects my body. You don't need to do this, because you're reading this book and I'm sharing some of the things I've learned. But if do you want to try this out, it's a good way to get in tune with your body.

...

Did you take some time to learn the above techniques? You've have had a lot of new concepts thrown at you. If you're used to hunching over a computer at work, learn to sit up straight and use your core when you get up and sit down.

If you stand at your job a lot, see if you can be more efficient when you walk from place to place. Try to keep your feet from getting tired by working on different muscles.

Go for a walk and practice out these techniques! Walk heel-toe, toe-heel, and pop. No one is watching you. No one at all.

Here's a benchmark to see if you've got the basics:
1) Can you feel where your center is at all times?
2) Can you feel good posture and bad posture?
3) Can you keep good posture while moving?
4) Do you know which method you'd been using to walk (before you started practicing heel-toe)?

...

At the very least, take two or three days and practice your posture and stepping heel to toe while moving your center. I'll wait.

These can be techniques you use the rest of your life! Taking a few days to learn them is worth it.

If you're sure you're ready to move on, here's one more check: can you successfully take a few steps heel-toe, in good posture, *while* moving your center with your motion?

If so, read on.

Ok. Now it's time to dive into something more subtle. Let's move on to using *both* legs while you walk. I bet you thought you were doing this already, but you probably weren't. At least not as well as you could. For example, do you walk slow or fast? If most people pass you as you walk, you can increase your speed by using both legs instead of just one to help yourself along. I'll explain what this means.

Let's do the example from the previous section. Stand straight, get a good connection in your center, one foot out in front, heel down, move your center forward, plant your foot, repeat. Got it? Good.

Let's add some more muscles into this. I want you to take a step as above and pause when your front foot hits the floor *while* your rear foot is still fully planted (with even the heel touching—no popping!). You should feel tension between your legs, or maybe a stretch in your back calf. From here, pull into the center of your body with the rear of your front thigh (your hamstrings on the stepping foot) and the front of your rear thigh (your quadriceps on the foot that will step next). You'll feel the pressure increase between your legs. Keep shifting your balance (your center) over your front foot and lift your back foot very slightly off the floor. It starts to swing forward on its own, doesn't it? That's good.

Try this again. Take one heel-toe step, plant both feet, squeeze your thighs together, release your back foot, and *as your back foot moves forward*, use this extra momentum to swing your new leg forward to plant it heel-toe in your next step.

Here's another important concept: as your rear foot swings forward, *now* is the time to release the tension in your thighs. If you keep this tension up it will restrict your movement rather than helping it, so it's important to relax in the middle of taking a step.

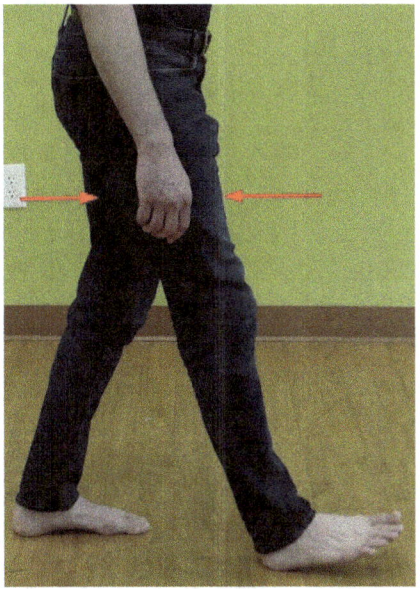

Figure 57: Use the muscles in both legs to walk, squeezing in along the red arrows before releasing your back foot from the floor.

Take a few minutes to practice and see if you can adapt the movement from jerky, stuttering steps to more fluid motion. Practice tensing, then relaxing your legs. If you need to, take out the walking part of this and pause in the middle of a step, with one leg in front of the other. Practice tensing your front hamstrings and rear quads, then release. Don't hulk out when you do it, just make a connection in your muscles. Do it ten or twenty times until you get the idea, even if it's not perfect. Once you've got that, come back here and read on.

> Tensing then relaxing afterward is a hard concept to practice and you probably won't get it right away. That's fine. Just keep it in mind as you continue working on using both legs to walk.

No really, go practice. You should be used to this by now.

Oh, and fix your posture. Yeah, I know.

...

Okay, ready to move on?

Now that you have the idea of this "step-squeeze-release-relax" motion, let's add yet *one more* layer of complexity (there's always one more...).

In the middle of your step, after you squeeze your thighs, as you release your rear foot from the floor, *keep* moving your hips (and thus your center) forward to the toes of your front foot. Your rear leg will move even farther forward. I know it sounds like I've already said this, but I promise it's different. The difference is subtle. You can check by looking straight down after the step. Your bellybutton should be directly between your feet, rather than at the toes of (what is now) your rear foot. If this sounds confusing, just try to walk and make sure you keep your center moving as you do it.

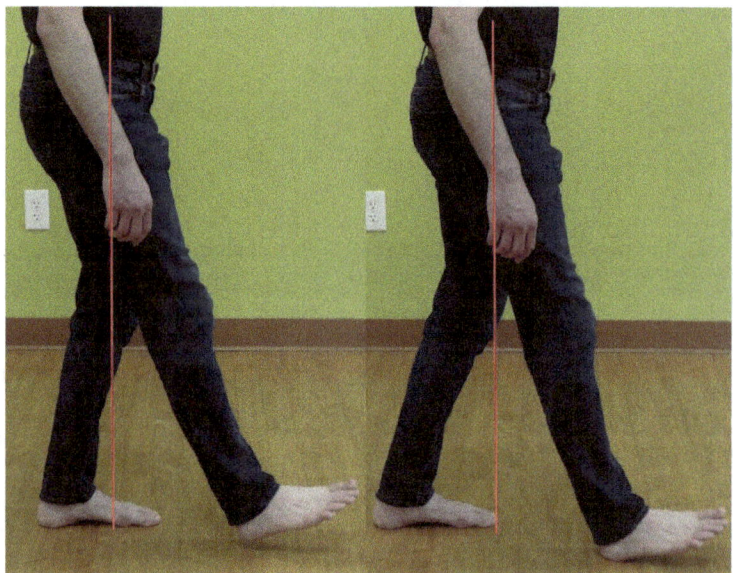

Figure 58: Left: stepping with the center of mass over the center of the back foot. Right: stepping with the center of mass over the toe of the back foot.

Go practice again, then come back so I can add one more detail (I told you there was always one more).

...

Okay, last time, really (for this section). Good posture, step forward heel-toe, squeeze your thighs, release, relax, move your center forward. Got all that? It's a lot to keep in your brain at once. Once you start to break this down to individual muscles, even very simple movements can turn out to be very complex. Your brain has learned over time how to do them without you thinking about them, and now you're breaking that pattern.

It can be frustrating to break things down like this, but I promise it will feel really good when you finally put it back together.

The final part is to keep moving your center forward even *past* your support foot as you swing your new leg out in front. Because if you move your center forward, you're going to have to compensate for the new placement by taking a larger step. This is the same thing you do when you start running, but we're doing it while you're walking. This means your walking stride is going to get longer, and you are going to take bigger steps. Thus, you will be able to walk faster. We're taking the mechanism of running and turning it into controlled walking!

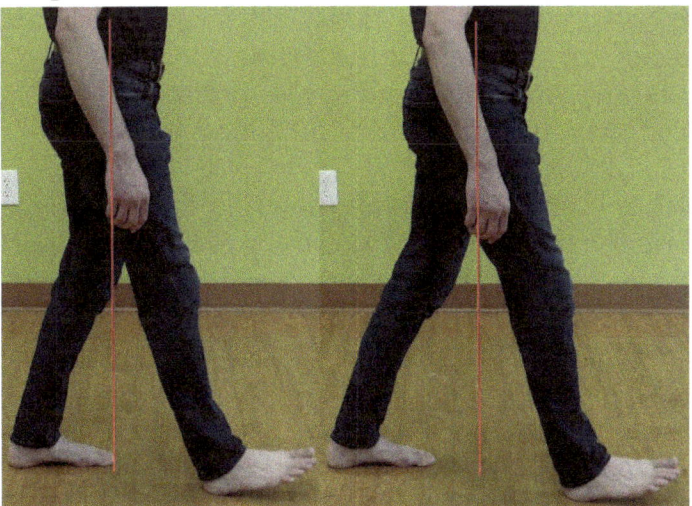

Figure 59: Left: stepping with the center of mass over the toe of the back foot. Right: Stepping with the center of mass past the toe of the back foot.

Throughout all this, remember your posture! You're likely looking down at your feet as you walk. Where's that bowling ball? Once you know where your center is going, pull your shoulders back and head up as you walk. Look directly forward, and you should have better control and balance.

Slowly speed your walk up as you get more comfortable with this long stride. Eventually, you'll be taking full, heel-toe steps and using both of your legs to propel your motion. Are you remembering your posture as you go faster? It's easy to bring your shoulders and head forward because that makes it seem like you're covering more ground. But resist that feeling. If you keep your head and shoulders above your center while you move, I promise you will actually be able to move faster. Even better, you will be able to stop, reverse, and change directions much quicker. This is helpful for not running into walls, or people, or tripping over pets with your new super speed. If that does become a problem, I have a handy section on falling at the end of this book.

Just like everything else, all this will take time to learn. It's all right to put this book down for a while and let your body process the changes you're making. There's a thing called muscle memory, which comes from doing an action so many times it's ingrained in the part of your brain that deals with reflexes rather than voluntary action. Athletes, musicians, or really anyone who does a repetitive task will find those processes moved to muscle memory. It's the same thing as learning to touch-type. When your fingers

All this may feel very mechanical as you practice, especially if you're feeling things out. That's fine to start. Try the motion, even if it feels clunky and robotic. Do each step as I've outlined, without blending them together yet. That comes later, after you're sure your muscles are operating in the correct manner and you've retrained your brain, just like any other sort of practice.

know where the keys are, you don't have to think about which one you're pressing.

There is a *lot* to unpack in this chapter—more than in the rest of the book to this point combined. It's okay to feel overwhelmed. It's okay to go back to a section and say, "I really didn't understand that part." Look at the pictures included with this book. They are another form of input and may make more sense than trying to digest a lot of words strung together.

Here are some tips and tricks to consider as you adapt your walking gait:

- The more you move your center forward while you take a step, the faster you will go. Eventually, you will turn the motion into running. Check this by running, then walking, to see the difference.

- Practice your posture and remember to keep up a connection while you walk. It's incredibly easy to forget. I do so on a regular basis, and I've been doing this for years. Always remember your hips, keeping them tucked, and keeping a connection to your core muscles. To check, you shouldn't be able to completely relax your abs while standing.

- See how fast you can walk while maintaining your motion and posture. Depending on your leg length, you may be able to take much bigger steps than you're used to. You also may hit the limit of how far your legs can comfortably reach. Always check that you can stop quickly and safely (within 1-2 steps) from a full walk!

- Make sure you don't overbalance and start to fall. You're learning to walk a second time, and you haven't done this since you were a toddler. Mistakes will happen! Check that your head is always above your center of mass.

Changing something so fundamental to how you move takes a lot of time to reprocess and relearn, and I've thrown a lot of information at you in this section. I know how hard it is, as I've had to relearn ingrained techniques several times while training in martial arts. It's never an easy process and can even take *years* to do. But change can also help you grow as a person. The key is dedication and remembering to go slowly while you learn. *Only* speed things up when you're sure you have the motion down. To test yourself, speed up to the point where something "breaks," that is, your posture goes, or you stumble, or something else. When you reach this point, you know you've gone too far and need to bring your speed down in order to get better at that motion. Practice some more, then speed things up again and see if you can go a little bit faster before things break. Pretty soon you'll be speed walking with the best of them!

Side issues in walking

Slumping

Yes, I've covered this a lot, but I want to reiterate the importance of posture, now you've read the most challenging parts. One of the most insidious and difficult-to-combat posture issues is slumping. I use this as a catchall term for the type of posture where you're sitting down, your neck is forward, and your stomach is hanging out. I'm not talking about whether you have a belly or flat abs, but whether your core is engaged, even if you're sitting down. Especially with the prevalence of office jobs, a lot of people nowadays sit for the better part of the day. When sitting for long periods of time, you want to relax, and that leads to letting the chair support you rather than sitting *up* in the chair.

But even when you relax, don't slump so the wrong muscles have to take up the slack. If you're standing up and tilting forward, your back structure has to compensate for lost posture, especially if you let your hips tip forward. The same thing applies in a chair, because if you slump, you are letting your hips disengage the connection in your abdomen. In this case, because your hips can't move anywhere, it's felt by your belly going soft and no longer holding your shoulders up. At this point, you start leaning forward, your neck juts out, and your shoulders roll forward. If you add to that holding a cell phone in

To clarify, I'm not saying you can never relax. You certainly can. Lean back in a chair, watch some TV, play a video game, listen to some music. Or when you're standing, lean against a wall and take a load off. But when you're actively engaged in an activity, try to keep your core engaged and your posture good. It might actually make you feel *more* relaxed when you relax!

your hand, it's very easy to lean your head forward so that you're looking down into your lap, thus exacerbating the problem.

Speaking of carrying things, what happens if your center moves backward (maybe carrying a backpack) or forward (such as being pregnant)? In this case, you might need to change your posture, especially if you don't have a choice where the extra load is (like pregnancy). In this case, you'll need to lean forward or backward to bring your upper body, which now contains the other object, over your new center. This is similar to lifting and carrying an object, which we'll go over in detail in the next section. For now, try to keep your good posture and connection while your upper body moves out of (unencumbered) alignment. You might need to tilt your head back or forward farther than you're used to!

In summary, it's always good to be aware of the posture I've discussed (ad nauseam) in this book. If you practice to the point where you know you have a connection all the way from your shoulders to your toes, you can keep that connection whether you're standing, carrying something, sitting, or lying down. Okay, I'll relent on that last one. You can relax when you're asleep.

As with everything else, be aware of what you're doing. If you start to encapsulate the lessons of this book, you may suddenly find you are aware when you're slumping. If you know you're doing something not good for your body, it's a lot easier to address the issue. That leads to the next topic.

Sitting Up and Sitting Down

As identified above, good posture is not limited to when standing up. It's also very important while you're sitting down. The posture and connection I've talked about have to become second nature, so much so that you maintain them in transitions as well, and not just while you are stationary.

Let's talk about one of the most common transitions, which is sitting down and standing back up. When you sit down, try not to flop into the chair you're sitting in. Instead, practice keeping the connection all the way down to the seat. It's going to feel a lot different, and it's going to take a little bit more musculature in your thighs.

Try it out now. I'll wait here.

How did sitting down feel? It always makes me feel very regal, as if I'm holding court while trying to sit down. This is, of course, because you're now doing it with correct posture and acting all refined.

> "Flopping" is a function of suddenly letting go of the connection between your hips and your shoulders, anticipating that the chair will take the load. If you simply don't have enough muscle to support yourself, try this: put both hands on your thighs and slide them to your knees as you sit down, pressing into your legs. This can make a connection that helps you keep your core engaged.

So, what about the other direction, when you want to stand back up? Do you bend forward so your shoulders come over the edge of the chair and sort of fall out of it until you can stand up? This is what most people do, but now you know about your center of mass, you know what's happening. When you lean your shoulders forward, you're moving your center of mass enough so it's now over your feet or your toes. Then it only takes a little bit of effort to stand up. This is all well and good, but don't make this a substitute for using the connection between your hips and your shoulders to help you stand.

Instead of rolling forward, keep that good posture and connection, and tilt your whole upper body forward. You still get the desired effect of changing your center of mass so it's over your feet and you can stand up. You'll also, again, use a little bit more muscle in your thighs to stand up. However, making a practice of this will also *increase* the muscle in your legs because you're using them more often.

Try these two methods out:

First, from a seated position, roll forward without good posture until you can "fall upward."

Next, keep your posture and lean forward before standing. If you need to, you can press your hands into your thighs to help push yourself up. If you have good posture, you may find it takes a much smaller shift to bring your shoulders forward to where you can stand up easily. And you thought walking was hard!

Walking on the Sides of Your Feet

Let's talk about less common aspects of people's walking gaits. The first is rolling your feet to the outside or inside while you walk. I don't have hard evidence to back this up, but I suspect if your feet rest more naturally at an open angle, you're more inclined to walk on the insides of your feet. On the other hand, if your toes tend to point toward each other at rest, you may be prone to walking on the outsides of your feet. Walking on the insides of your feet, to me, is the more ergonomically worrying position. When you do this, your knees have a tendency to buckle inward, which can cause strain on the tendons and ligaments in that area. There is also little musculature support on the inside of your foot where the arch is.

Remember I said way back in the anatomy section that I would be talking later about moving on the sides of your feet? This still isn't it!

Walking on the outside of your foot is also something to be avoided, if possible. This puts strain on the outside of the knee rather than inside, although you have more support because you can still use your toes to grip the floor. There are some martial arts stances that actually have you stand on the "ridge edge" of your feet. Walking this way all the time, however, means you must divert extra effort to keeping your balance.

Wobbling

There are several different ways people wobble to the sides when they walk rather than moving forward in a straight line. Often, it's when people are taking their ease, and simply not walking very fast, enjoying the view. The tendency here is to shift your body over one foot and then over the other, as this diverts momentum from going forward and makes you slow down. I'm not as concerned about this one, as it does sort of make sense. You don't have any particular place to be, and you aren't concerned about being incredibly efficient while you walk. That's fine.

> There may be reasons to wobble while walking. Just be aware that every time you shift your body to the side rather than shifting forward, you're decreasing your walking efficiency.

There are some other forms of wobbling that seem to be more of a habit for people. Moving your shoulders side to side, or one shoulder forward then the other, while you walk seems intimidating. You are swaggering or showing off that you're in control. But to do this all the time when you're trying to get somewhere is counterintuitive. You waste a lot of energy doing so, and you are less stable on your feet. If you *were* trying to intimidate someone, you're actually *more* susceptible to being pushed over!

Finally, if you keep your weight too far backward while you walk (so that your center is more than that two fingers behind your bellybutton), then you're going to fall into a sort of swaying rhythm, where your hips move over one foot then the other while you walk. Again, this keeps you from moving forward as efficiently as you could.

Head Bobbing

This last issue is concerned with connection, but not between your hips and your shoulders. It's the connection between your shoulders and your head. You may see people do this, or may even have done it yourself, where you walk almost like a pigeon, bobbing your head forward with every step. If you follow the good posture like I covered throughout this book, your ears are going to be over your shoulders. If this is the case, then you shouldn't be able to bob your head forward. If you let your head fall forward or are looking at a cell phone in your hand for example, your head may start to bob simply from the up-and-down motion of walking. It's fairly easy to correct this if you reset to a good posture: ears over your shoulders, shoulders back, hips tucked, knees slightly bent, feet straight in front of you.

> You are not a velociraptor. Don't head bob while you're walking, as if looking for prey (or a cell signal). Hold your cellphone up higher, if needed.

I am certain there are many more side issues I could get into, but this is all I'm going to cover for now. Mainly because we have another half of your body to cover! If you've practiced everything to this point, you'll have a good handle on keeping your posture steady, keeping your core engaged, and moving your center forward while you walk. Keep practicing those principles in the lower half of your body while supporting your top half. It's time to get into more fun things you can do while learning how to operate your body!

How to Pick up Chicks (and Dudes)!

We just investigated walking stride and how you can affect it, as well as how to move your center with your step. The upper body is a little different. First, it doesn't include your center of mass, as I mentioned before, and second, it depends on the stability of your lower body's resistance against whatever you're standing on. If you're sitting or lying down, you'll depend dramatically less on your lower body, but that also limits your range of motion and what you can manipulate.

However, the same warnings apply! If you haven't practiced your posture, or skipped over the arm anatomy, go back and read it now. I'll still be here. We're going to be doing detailed manipulation from here on, and the more you're in tune with your body, the easier it will be (and the less likely you are to hurt yourself).

Let's start with some simpler concepts and exercises, and move to more complex ones afterward. A lot of what I'll discuss here depends on using the lower body as well as the upper for maximum strength and mechanical advantage, but I will add some modifications for those whose lower bodies are argumentative or apathetic.

> Think of the lower half of your body as the stable base, which contains your center and supports your weight. In contrast, your upper body is the dexterous half that interfaces with other objects. Of course, if you stand on your hands, this will be reversed...

Heavy Thoughts

Humans have a unique structure in the animal kingdom. We're fully bipedal and made to walk or stand that way for long periods of time. While there are lots of other animals that can operate bipedally, and many birds are fully bipedal as well, only humans walk with their head completely above their center of mass. Remember the experiment with the bowling ball? You are out of correct alignment if your head is forward like any other animal or bird. This posture comes from humans having an extra curve in their spine—that lower back or lumbar area that hurts so often. That's one of the tradeoffs of bipedalism.

There are a lot of works that address *why* humans are bipedal, so I'm not going to cover that question here. After all, this is called *How* to Operate Your Body. Instead, I'm going to show you *how* bipedalism gives you some really excellent opportunities to use your arms. Let's start with the one that is again somewhat unique to humans: lifting. Lifting objects itself is not new to the animal kingdom, but most animals use their jaw, or maybe their feet, trunk, or in rare cases, hands. The jaw is an incredibly powerful muscle, even in humans, but not one we often use, given the choice between hands and mouth. We have (usually) two appendages right in front of us that grip, manipulate, and carry with high reliability and dexterity. We don't have to put things down to walk, like birds do when using their feet as hands, and we don't have to put an object down to eat or talk, like animals that use their mouths do. Finally, because we're built for long-distance walking, we can continue to carry objects as long as our endurance lets us, compared to even other primates, who will eventually have to go back to all fours on the ground or in the trees, losing that opportunity to carry.

How do you carry an object? The first stage is before you even approach it. You eye it up, and mentally gauge if you can even lift it. Humans are *really* good at this. We make assumptions on how an object lands or rolls, what size it is, what it's made out of, and other clues. Then we go in for the lift. This is how you can tell that a "heavy" prop in a movie or play is actually made of Styrofoam, or why you might get tripped up when you pick up a box you assume is filled with hardback books and it turns out that's the one with paper towels (or vice versa)!

> There is at least one study supporting the hypothesis that great apes can gauge weight like we can:
> https://pmc.ncbi.nlm.nih.gov/articles/PMC

Approach

The first part of lifting is a combination of *kinesthesia* and *proprioception*, two fun words that mean, respectively, the awareness of the movement and direction of *your* body, and the awareness of the position and posture of your body *in respect to* the position and weight of objects *around* your body. All that to say: as a human, you're pretty good at gauging how to approach an object and interact with it.

To break those two fancy words into more useful parts: what happens when you start to interact with an object, especially a heavy one? You want to know how close you are to it, how much it weighs, how far you have to reach to get it, if you need to pull it toward you, where its position is relation to your center of mass (and whether you're standing, sitting, or lying down), and whether you can grip it with one hand, two hands, or some other method.

All this passes through your mind in a fraction of a second. This is why the Boston Dynamics robots are still a good way away from effectively carrying objects bipedally. They're getting pretty good at the kinesthesia part (how the robot body moves), but once they start interacting with other objects, the difficulty of controlling such robots goes up exponentially because of proprioception (the feedback of the body touching another object).

Let's look at approaching objects that take two hands to carry. First, how do you know you need two hands? It's a complex equation of where the center of the balance is, how bulky it is, how big it is compared to the stretch of your hand, and simply how much it weighs. If there's an object that falls between one hand and two hands for manipulation, we might attempt to pick it up with one hand (often followed by an "oops, that won't work"), then use both when we've determined it's on the *two* hands side of the equation.

> Look around and eye up objects around you. I bet you can tell at a glance which need two hands and which only need one. Your eyes might even pause for a moment on those objects in between while you calculate.

Balance is an important part of this evaluation, both for your body and for the object. Try this: pick up any sort of object around you with one hand: a phone, a water bottle, a pen, a laptop or heavy book... How close do you naturally get to the center of mass when you pick it up? Does it feel like there's an even amount of weight on either side of your hand? How about something like a pen? Do you pick it up from one end or the other? No, you normally pick it up from the middle, or maybe toward the weightier end if it has a big cap. You reach for the center of mass, so that it's easy to pick up and manipulate.

Here's another exercise. If you have a couple similar refillable water bottles around, fill one all the way up with water, and the other only about a third of the way full. Have someone else mix them up while you close your eyes, then reach blindly for one of them with one hand. Where do you pick it up? How long passes after you touch it that you can determine how full it is, and thus where the center of mass is? It might be sooner than you think.

When you need two hands, often the deciding factor is weight or size. An object might be light, but simply too big to pick up with one hand, like a big empty box or a yoga ball. Or the center might be liable to change drastically if you pick it up with one hand, like a container with liquid.

A consideration I haven't talked about yet with lifting objects is whether it needs to stay in the same orientation after you're holding it. Two hands are much more effective at balancing the load and keeping an object steady. We'll talk about precision and dexterity in the next section.

All said, there's a lot you innately consider when first coming into contact with an object you plan to pick up. But what happens when the object is very heavy or unwieldy?

Brace Your Support

We're going to switch gears for a moment and look back at what your body is doing while you're reaching out with grabby hands for whatever you want to pick up. How far away is it and how high is it compared to your center? That's going to have a big effect on how your body is positioned, and whether you're on your way to injuring something.

Let's go back to the bowling ball example because a) it's the size and weight of your head, b) it's a heavy thing you need to hold with two hands, and c) who doesn't own their own bowling ball? Where do you naturally hold a bowling ball (or any heavy, two-handed object)? Most likely, you hold a heavy object right in front of your stomach. It's comfy and your arms naturally bend that way.

But *before* you get to that point, you must bring the object

Have you made the mistake of trying to carry a flat object with liquid on it? The center of mass of a body of water is fluid (pun intended) so it's hard for us to control where it slops, and we usually make a mess.

to you, and this is where injuries happen. When I worked at a large construction company, there was a weight limit of 35 lbs (16 kg) on what a person could safely lift without an assisting device. This is equivalent to about three human heads (or bowling balls), if you're keeping track. Now while this doesn't seem like a whole lot compared to what we lift on an everyday basis, it's important to take into account not only how much an object weighs, but how far it is away from you.

The torque (rotational force) put on your back (and other parts of your body) is equal not just to the weight of the thing you're picking up, but the weight times the distance it is away from your center of mass. So that bowling ball held right in front of your stomach seems to weigh about a fourth as much as a bowling ball held at arm's length. Plus, the force is going through your arm and shoulder, rather than directly into your center. It's putting about four times the amount of strain on the thing that is resisting the weight which, in most cases, is your spine.

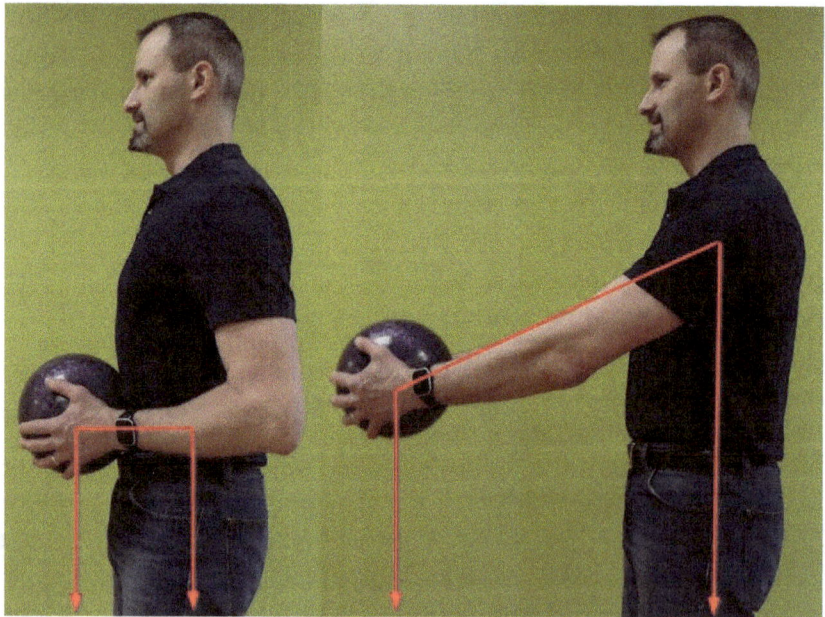

Figure 60: The change in effort required to hold an object close to your center and at arm's length

All this to say, when you are reaching out to pick up a heavy object, think about how that weight is suddenly going to act on your spine once *you* are the only thing supporting it. Some good options are:

1) Pull the object closer, if it's sitting on something solid, so that it's closer to your center.

2) Test the weight to make sure it's only as heavy as you assumed it was.

3) Raise or lower your center so it matches the position of the object.

4) Brace your back or legs against a firm structure so that the force doesn't only act on your spine.

The first and second options should be pretty self-explanatory. The third one we're going to cover in an upcoming section, and the fourth option is a little more complex. It could be hooking your foot on something, leaning on a ladder, or even lifting while using a mobility device. When you do this, you still need to have good posture. If your back is straight, the force will go into your legs and into the object. If your back is bent, the force will act on your spine. This is similar to walking with a backpack or while pregnant, which I covered in the previous section. You're connecting with another object, which we'll also talk about in the "Carrying" and "Body Mechanics" sections. For now, let's get to those grabby hands.

> Why does bracing work? Because you're changing where your center of mass is. You're now "attached" to another object (just like when you're wearing a backpack) and its center and your center can be treated as one!

Engage

So now you've got your hot little hands on an object. What do you do with it? Human hands are very dexterous. You can grasp with the palm of your hand (with either the "standard" grip or the "crab" grip), you can pinch between your thumb and any other fingertip, you can pinch in any of the three spaces between fingertips, and you can even do a combination of these things to pick up multiple objects at one time. How often have you had to grab up a bunch of items when leaving the house in a hurry, or passing through a metal detector, or simply trying to carry too many things at once like an overwrought claw machine?

That forearm rotation between your radius and ulna provides a lot of options when lifting. For "picking up," you'll likely turn your palm down and grasp with the tips of your fingers or maybe the palm if it's a heavy item. Generally, this type of lifting puts more stress on the shoulder, which limits the amount of weight we can lift this way, using only the grasping forearm muscles, the biceps, and the triceps.

> The difference between "picking up" and "lifting" is mostly palm and elbow position. Try picking up a water bottle from the top. Your elbow is pointed out, your palm down. Pick it up (or "lift" it) from the base and your elbow points down, your palm up or sideways.

Try this exercise: can you pick up a pen or a pencil between your ring finger and pinky, or between your middle and ring finger, and *then* pick up another writing utensil with forefinger and thumb? On top of that, can you write with the pen or pencil between your thumb and forefinger? Can you then switch the positions of the writing implements and write with the other one, all with one hand? I bet you can. Human hands are pretty nimble. Bonus points if you can also uncap a pen with that same hand before you write with it.

However, for "lifting," turning the palms up gives you a lot of stronger options that start to engage your biceps, triceps, shoulders, and down into your back and even your legs. There are a lot of surfaces you can use for this action. While it doesn't have as much dexterity as picking things up, you can lift with pretty much any surface from your fingertips to elbows, then depending on your starting stance, even with your upper arms and shoulders. This is how waiters can carry five plates down one arm and pass them out to customers like dealing playing cards.

Balance is an intricate part of lifting (and good posture helps balance!), if you aren't actively gripping the object with your fingers to keep it from falling. Take an object (preferably non-breakable) and rest it on your forearm. Can you keep it from falling off? Try something grippy, but rigid, like a phone with a rubberized phone case (maybe only a few inches over another surface...). Now try something rigid and smooth, like a book or water bottle. Finally try something floppy, like a towel, pillow, or maybe even a computer hand rest. They will all take a differing amount of control to keep from falling off, but you can likely hold all the objects, at least for a few seconds.

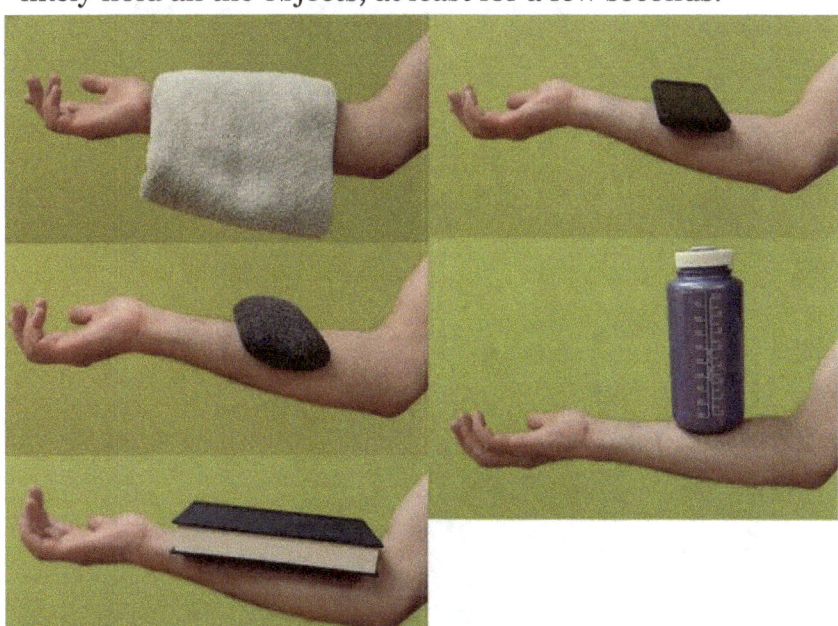

Figure 61: The forearm has a lot of lifting potential!

And since we're talking about forearm manipulation, what about those other great gripping surfaces: the elbow and armpit? Because you've got two manipulators out in front of you while you're bipedal, you can pinch between the elbow and your side, and you can also fold your arm in and pinch between forearm and biceps. There's not nearly as much dexterity here, but there's a tradeoff with how much strength you have, especially because this is closer to your center. The same thing, though smellier, applies to your armpit. It's a great place to tuck an object while you need both hands free to manipulate something else.

Speaking of gripping surfaces, the wrist is another great one, close to your fingers, and nimbler than your elbows and shoulders. Try pinning something against your side with your wrist while you use your fingers for another task. You can still get a lot done.

Of course, now I'm imagining someone with two or three pens in each hand, wrists holding papers against their sides, a water bottle and wallet in their elbows and a book under each arm...

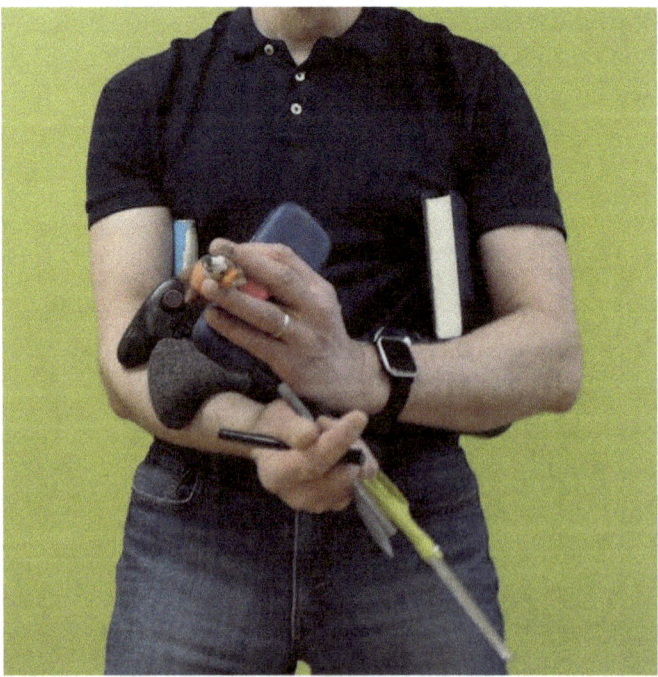

Figure 62: You can hold a lot of things at once!

To add to this, you can actually change how your arms are connected to your body! It's all a matter of joints. For lifting, it's easier to move a heavy object with your whole body than with just your arms. So, if you make a connection between your elbows and your stomach (very near your center of mass) then suddenly your lifting ability grows. Refer back to Figure 60, then try out this example.

Find an object that is *heavy* for you. A kettlebell, a dumbbell, a jug of liquid, that convenient bowling ball... Now grip it in the best way you can with both hands. Keep about a fist-width of distance between your elbows and your sides. First, move the object up and down slowly in front of you. Feel what's engaging as you do this. Generally, if you go higher than your center and chest, more weight is put on your shoulders. Slightly lower and there's weight on your pectoral muscles. Lower still and you'll feel it low in your pectorals and in your abdominals.

> The more you lock out your joints and remove them from the lifting circuit, the stronger you are. Joints are amazingly versatile, but they are also weak points.

Now adjust your connection point. Plant your elbows on your sides and keep them touching. You won't be able to lift the object much past your chest, but that's ok. In your new range of motion with your elbows on your sides, you should feel much less weight from the object. That's because it's going through your center of mass and you're short-circuiting the force straight from your elbows to your abs and back, which are much stronger. This is a good way to get a forearm workout too!

What if you do need to lift this object higher? Try this. As you raise the object, your elbows will want to come away from your sides. Instead, try to slide your elbows around your front and, if you're flexible enough, press them together in front of you as you lift. Now you can raise with both arms stuck together, which again diminishes the feeling of the total weight. If you need to lift this heavy object even higher, eventually your elbows will have to separate too, but you can try to keep your wrists touching! Whenever you make a circuit between the halves of your body—feet, hands, arms, and legs—you have more strength and control in the limbs that are touching. We'll cover this again briefly in the body mechanics section.

Lifting With the Whole Body

Let's keep on talking about objects that are heavy. When you encounter these, you'll need to incorporate more of your body to offset the weight of the object. This helps avoid putting that weight on your joints and causing them injury or simply falling over. It comes down to the adage you've likely heard hundreds of times: "lift with your legs." But let's break it down a bit.

We talked about lifting above your center, but what happens when the heavy object is low to the ground, and you need to get under it to lift? Along with your arms, let's incorporate your core and legs into the mix. In the section on the knees, I go over how to properly perform a squat. If you haven't (yet) read that section, then briefly, keep your feet shoulder-width apart, tuck your hips under you and get to your good posture. Then stick your butt out as you bend your knees so your center stays more or less over your heels as you squat down. Better yet, go back and read that section. Remember, it's okay to take a break from the concepts in this book to give them time to sink in.

How does squatting help you lift? Because for getting under the object with your arms, you don't want to bend over and expose your back to a very long lever arm from your shoulder to the object below you. Remember the section on bracing? We're affixing another object to our body and changing our center. That same multiplication of torque still works if the distance you're reaching is *down*, not *out*. However, you can't slide an object up through the air to you like you can with one sitting on a flat surface. You'll need to bring your center to it.

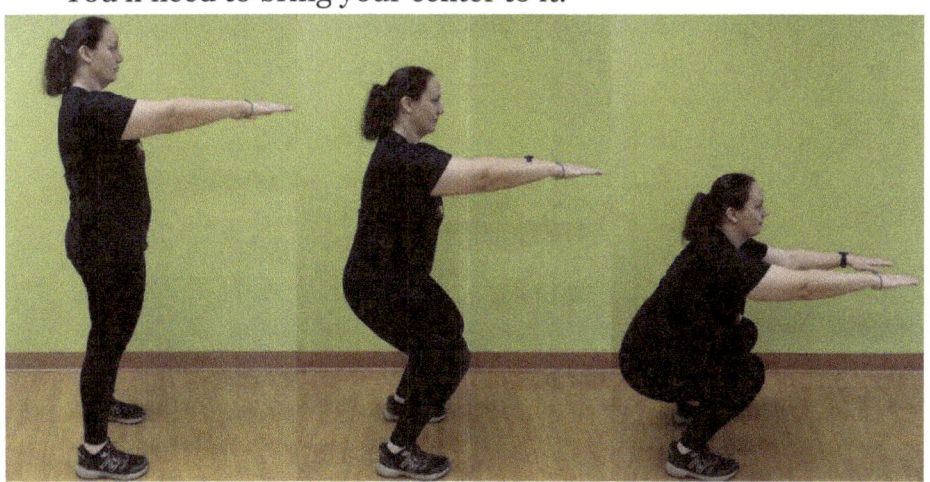

Figure 63: A properly performed squat.

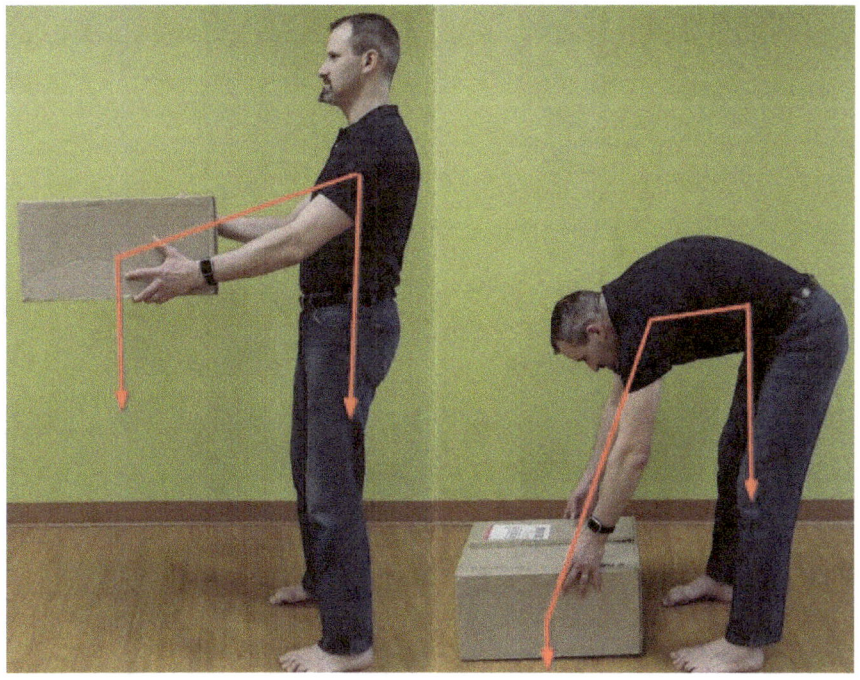

Figure 64: The torque multiplication of picking up a box without lowering your center might be as bad or worse than holding a box out in front of you.

This is where you get to do your workout at the same time as lifting that object. Do a squat! And do it in good form. If the heavy object is very low (and you can squat past 90 degrees) you can do a full squat in order to lift it up. Engage with the object with those graspers, and tuck your elbows into your sides to immobilize your elbow joints like we talked about last section. Even better, you'll want to tense your abs and back muscles so the connection (remember your posture!) in your body goes all the way from your fingertips and right down to the floor. We'll cover even more about making that connection immovable in the more advanced section on using your core.

Now you're at the low point of your (correct posture) squat, your hands or forearms are firmly attached to the object, and your elbows are as close to your sides as they can get. If they can't touch your sides because you have to reach for the object, bring them toward your center as close and as soon as you can, once the object is in the air. Reverse your squat and stand up. Keep good posture along the way and keep your head up. Once you're standing, keep those elbows tucked and the object close to your belly. You'll be able to hold an object that might normally be too heavy for you.

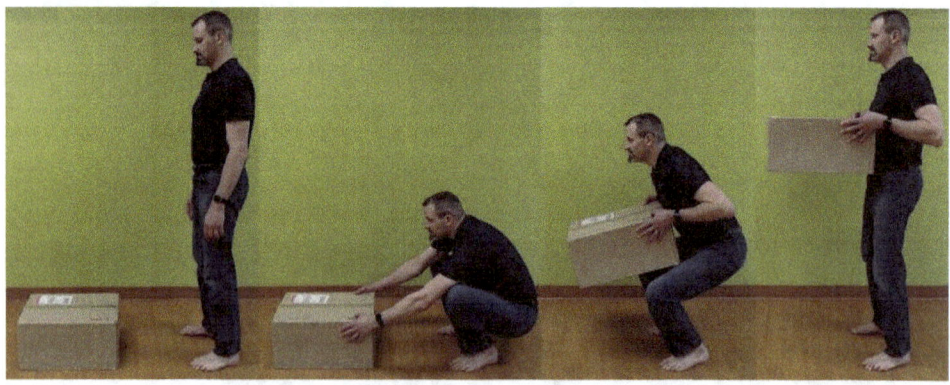

Figure 65: Lowering your center to lift an object.

Carrying for Long Distances

Congratulations, you have a heavy (or bulky) object! Now what do you do with it? Presumably you want to put it somewhere else. What if that somewhere is far away? You're going to have to carry it there.

If you've read this book in order, you now know how to walk correctly. I'll assume your walking posture and stride are a thing of beauty, and you keep your head up regally the whole time. If not, maybe go back and touch on that section again.

If you have a bulky or heavy object you need to transport more than a step or two, the best thing to do is pretend like that object is now an essential part of your body and you can't live without it. Hold it close like a lover and never let it go (except when you need to set it down). Tuck your elbows into your sides so the object is right at your center. Try to find a natural "ridge" with your pants, belt, belly, what have you, around that area and "seat" the object firmly there. Tense your abs so they press into the object. This, in effect, moves your center slightly closer to the object. Feel as if they become one. You and this object are going on a journey together.

If that doesn't work for whatever reason, lay the object across your chest or over your shoulder. Try to have it touch as much surface area as possible while you're carrying it. We can accommodate heavy objects much easier if they're touching our bodies, and especially if they are close to or in front of our center. The less we have to move our posture out of alignment, the better. This, of course, is an issue if the heavy thing you're carrying is especially hot, cold, spiky, poisonous, corrosive, or any other

> Remember walking with a backpack or while pregnant in the previous section? This is the same concept. Your center will move a little, and your (good) posture will adjust so you still keep your head above your center.

uncomfortable conditions. If so, protective gear might be in order.

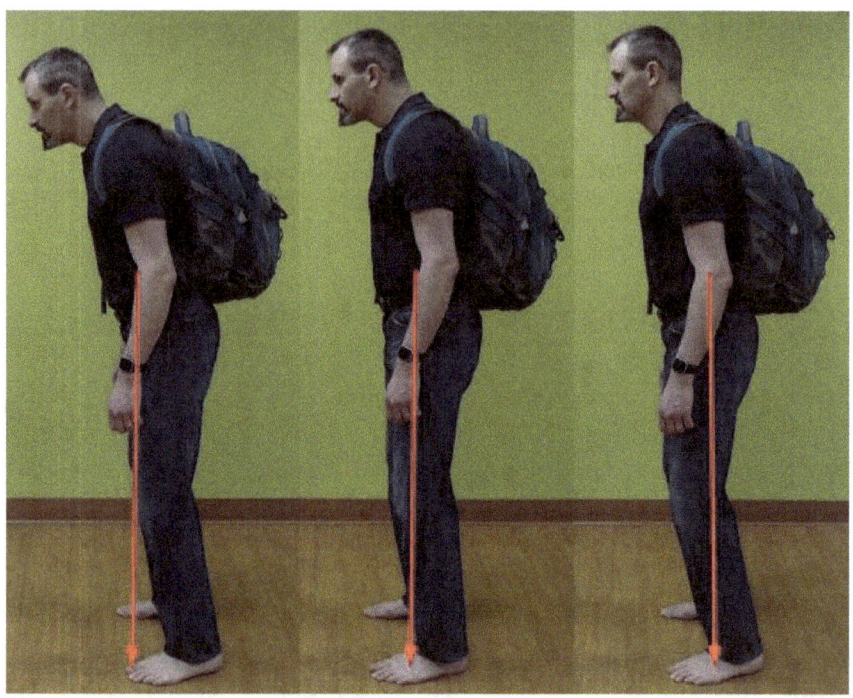

Figure 66: When moving or standing with a heavy object attached to you, try not to lean forward (left), or put your head forward (middle). Instead try to adjust your stance to compensate with good posture for the change in your center (right).

Fortunately, humans are endurance hunters. Researchers looking at the muscle makeup of humans vs. animals found most animals have around 66% fast-twitch muscle content (muscles that activate quicker, but also fatigue quicker) and 33% slow-twitch (muscles that are better for endurance, but don't activate as fast). Humans, on the other hand, have about 30% fast twitch and 70% slow twitch, which means we can't move as fast in short bursts, but can keep going for much longer. We've

You can find an article summarizing the results here: https://www.science.org/content/article/how-chimps-outmuscle-humans

traded overall strength for increased dexterity. Even animals with grasping hands, like primates, racoons, and rodents don't have the same range of dexterity we do. The only other animal with a similar percentage muscle breakdown is the slow loris, a sleepy nocturnal primate. Make of that what you will with respect to humans...

Returning to the original (tongue-in-cheek) title for this section, these principles can be used on more malleable objects as well as rigid ones. Lifting up a person is much like lifting up a large box (except you need to ask permission). You already know about where the center of mass is for a person. There's no reason you can't pick up another human that weighs about as much or less than you do. Just make sure they're alright with it.

If they're standing, this is very similar to lifting a box. Approach the other person side-on, with one foot on either side of them. Set your stance, bend your knees, and first get your center of mass *below* theirs. If they are shorter than you, you may need to squat down a lot. Just like everything else we've been talking about, joints are great places to maneuver yourself and others. Now you're down low, hook the arm to the person's front under their knees and hook the other arm around their waist. This way they can settle back as in a chair. That's you. You're now the chair.

Remember to only lean forward enough to keep your head over your (new) center! Keep good posture and try to lift straight up with your legs, while gluing your elbows to your sides. The other person can put their hands around your neck to support themself and help balance.

You can come at this a different way if the other person is bigger than you and you don't think you'll be able to support lifting them directly up. This is again using the power of your center.

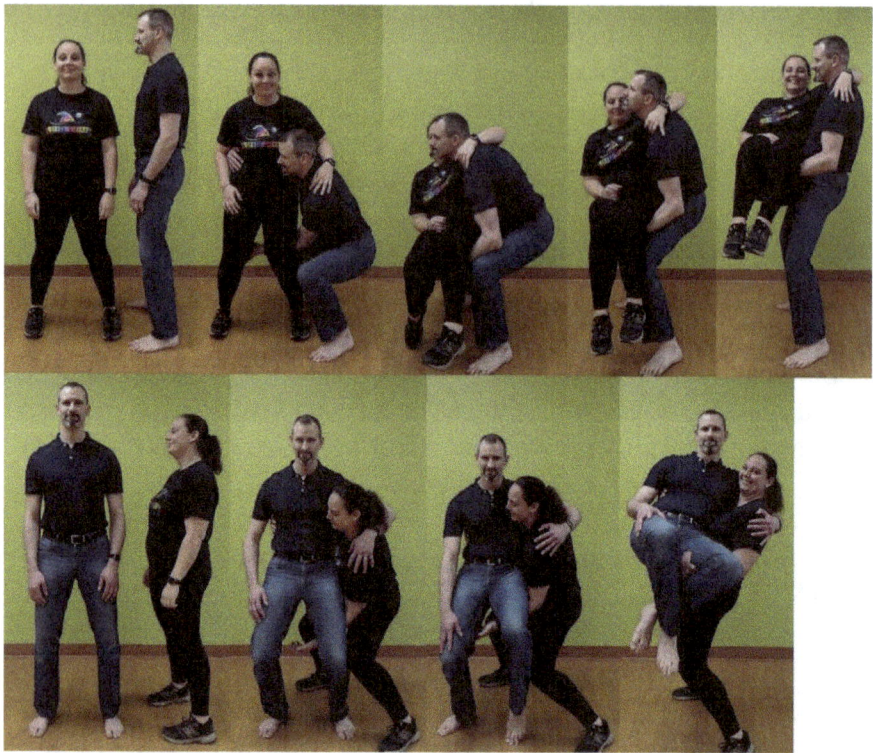

Figure 67: Lifting another person in a "chair" carry. Note how the center adjusts for the added forward weight.

Start almost the same way as before, except this time the person who will be carried is facing *your* side, not the other way around. Step between their legs with the foot closest to them, grasp their arm, and duck your head underneath so it's over your shoulder. At the same time, you should be keeping good posture and squatting down. Again, you want to make certain your center is below theirs, the lower the better.

Once down here, use the backs of their knees again as a manipulation point. Move in so your shoulder is underneath their pelvis, and lift with your knees, moving the other person across your shoulders as you do. Still try to keep your posture, with back straight, and neck not leaning too far forward. Just like any other heavy object, the more their weight (concentrated in their center) is right above *your* center, the easier it will be to lift them. From here, continue to straighten up with the other person draped across your shoulders like an ungainly feather boa.

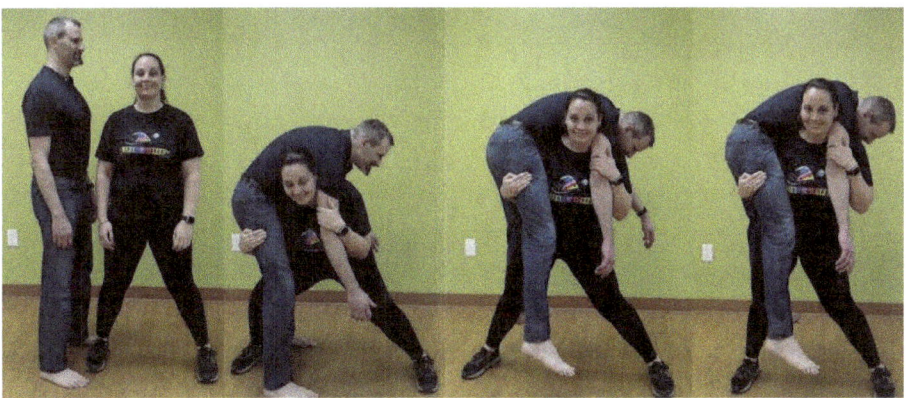

Figure 68: Lifting another person in a "fireman" carry. This is especially useful if the person is taller than you.

Congrats! You have a person. Now what? Presumably you've lifted them up for some reason, perhaps even to carry them somewhere important quickly.

Fortunately, we've covered how to walk already, though if you are carrying something close to your own weight, remember your center changes how you move with that load.

First, make sure your posture is as good it can be with a human lying across your shoulders. Adjust your head so it's over your new center. If your new center is farther back, you want to move your head back, and vice versa.

Second, be very deliberate in how you walk, making sure to completely plant each foot heel to toe before putting your weight (and your plus one) on that foot as you take another step. If you've walked like a penguin on ice, this is a similar concept. You're keeping your center more directly under you than if you're simply walking freely. This is the opposite of how you would move your center over your front foot when trying to walk faster.

Finally, be very careful of how you turn and reach with this other person. Their weight is directly on top of your spine, but twisting or adjusting them quickly could cause injury, just like trying to lift a heavy object that's at the extent of your arm's reach. We'll cover how to reduce the possibility of injuring yourself in the section about the core!

Just like in the section on walking, there's a lot of information in these pages. These exercises deal with manipulation of other objects, rather than propelling yourself, so you're not changing as many of your habits here. It's still good to take some time and go over these actions again until they make sense. Feel out how your body changes as you move objects around! The more you're comfortable with using your whole body to augment your arms while you lift, the less likely you are to injure something while lifting.

And that's how you pick up chicks (and dudes)!

Body Mechanics Tips and Tricks

In this section, I'm going to go over a bunch of tips and tricks that are generally useful, but rely on knowing about your anatomy and how to use your arms and legs. So by this point, if you haven't gone through the sections on anatomy, how to walk, and how to lift things, I'd highly advise reading through them first. Some of these techniques use your arms, some use your legs. We're also going to do a deep dive into how to use your core! Even if you don't fully understand these ways of moving, let them percolate through your brain and see if any of them stick, or help you out in the future.

Fast and Loose vs. Slow and Steady Movement

The temptation when you're able to move more efficiently is to also move faster. This is not always the best plan, as the faster you move, the more you lose the posture and muscular connection you've been trying to develop.

When you're learning a new skill, remember to start out slowly. Even if you feel silly, or aren't progressing as fast as somebody else, there's no reason to compare yourself against others. If you can do a skill just as well slowly as you can fast, then you're well on your way to mastering it.

I always tell my martial arts students I would rather see a form performed slowly and correctly rather than fast and sloppily. When you move slowly, you are

If you've ever practiced a musical instrument or other physical activity, you're probably aware of how making slow movements and speeding up can lead to better results than trying to learn at a faster speed.

also able to weed out inbuilt inefficiencies that are hard to see when you move fast. The total learning time may end up being *shorter* than if you go fast and mess things up. Keep in mind as you move about life that *fast is not always the best option*. Better if you start out slow and work on a skill until you're able to do it either slow or fast.

Muscles Moving Against Each Other

Your muscles don't move in isolation. Since you suspend yourself vertically and against gravity while standing, you naturally use some muscles more than others, especially when you stand up. As Newton said, "For every action there is an equal and opposite reaction." This means when you push against something, that something will push back against you. This is also true inside your body.

When you push with one arm, there's going to be a reaction, and if you don't balance yourself, you'll turn in a circle. You already know how to compensate, but we can take this concept and turn it into an advantage rather than simply resisting gravity.

I covered this concept briefly in the sections on connection and isometrics, but I wanted to expand on the topic now you've gone through the rest of the exercises. I'm going to give you some examples about using muscular tension to offset everyday actions.

Try this: stand in front of an open doorway, and push with one hand into one side of the doorframe. You can feel the stress all the way down your legs into the ground, because you're compensating for not rotating away from the doorframe where you pushed it. Now put one hand on either side of the doorframe and push equally. You only need to resist the backward motion. Obvious, right? Let's try a more complicated example.

Go back to that same doorway, and this time hook just your fingers around the doorframe so you can pull yourself to one side. If you only pull with one hand, then you have to resist being pulled over. Now let's do the same second part as before. Wrap the fingers of one hand around either side of the doorframe. If you pull equally with both hands, you stay where you are, and as a bonus, the rest of your body doesn't have to resist falling over. Muscles are moving against each other to keep you in place. You can put as much force as you want to into one hand and still resist that force with the other hand. Newton is proven correct once again.

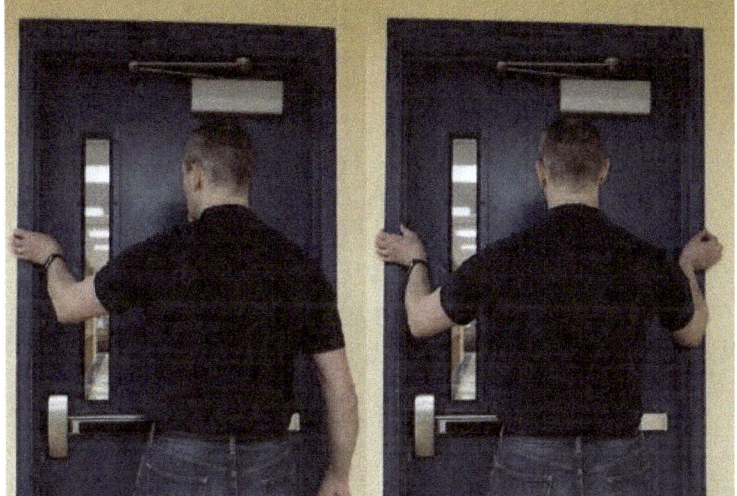

Figure 69: Pulling with one side of the body (left) vs. both sides of the body (right). Note the center has to move to adjust for the force.

I know these seem like silly examples, but I want you to understand the idea because this is a sort of nebulous concept. Let's try something more complex. Say you're trying to hammer a nail into a wall. If you stand completely still and try to move the hammer only with your forearm, you're only going to get so much force out of it. Feel free to try this, but please find a safe and inconspicuous surface first. Don't blame this book for holes in your walls.

Once you've got the idea, try hammering again, but this time let your upper body move with the motion so that your off shoulder (the one you're not using to hammer with) starts moving as well. Because you are now moving both sides of your body, you can coordinate the timing so that you get much more force in each hammering motion. It's sort of a whip-like action, passing through your upper body.

How about a less...destructive example? Say you're getting food out of the fridge and setting it on the counter. You either open the fridge with your dominant hand and pick up the item with your non-dominant hand, or vice versa. Now you have two things you need to do: you need to put the food down somewhere, and you also need to close the fridge.

> I guess you technically don't have to have good posture for this, but I hope you do after reading the rest of this book.

Rather than make this two separate actions, make it the same action. Use the action that requires more force—closing the fridge—as a counterbalance to get your body moving in the right direction to put the food down on the counter. Rather than waste energy moving one direction, then moving in another direction, use Newton's action and reaction to reposition yourself where you need to be. When you push the door closed, let that force aid you in moving away from it toward your destination.

However, in order to do so, you must have a good connection through your body and core. That way, you're not wasting energy by twisting your body, when you could be using that energy to swing a foot in the direction you want to go. I could go on this topic for a long time, as it ties in strongly with what I teach in my martial arts class. For now, try redirecting energy into the next action that you do.

Completing a Circle

Let's move on to the concept of completing a circle with your body. It's related to moving your muscles against each other. If you can create a circle with your limbs, you're able to use more of the maximum strength of your body.

Here's an easy example. Try to lift a heavy object with one arm. Now add the other arm to it, even without adding its full strength. You can simply touch your arm with one finger of the other hand. You may suddenly be able to lift the object. It's the same idea as if you try to steady a hand that's doing a precise action, by touching it with your other hand.

On the physical side, if you use both halves of your body in an action, it becomes easier to balance, or to offset the weight of the object you're dealing with.

The combination of this physical and mental feedback means you're better able to compensate for any errors while you do whatever it is you're doing.

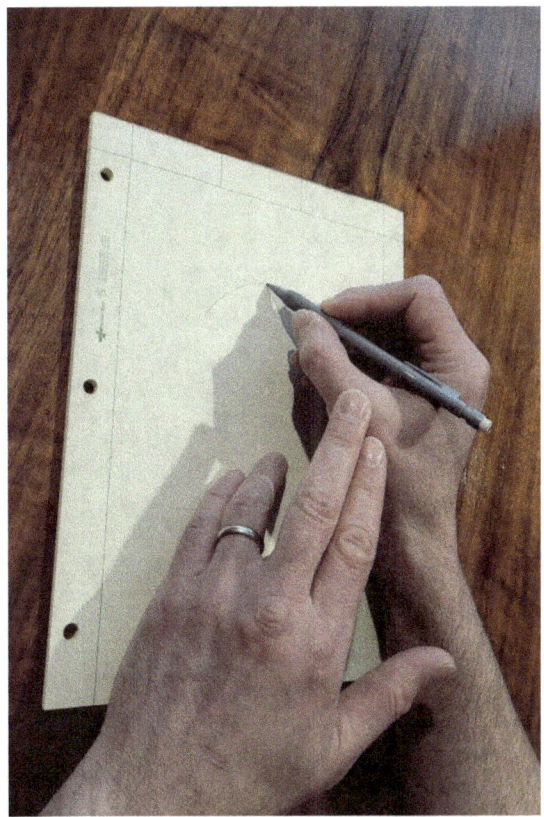

Figure 70: Touching one side of your body to the other can give greater fine control of action.

I'm not going to go deep into the mechanical reasons behind this, but I believe it has to do with your kinesthetic sense. That is, knowing where your limbs are. If you have two limbs occupied in the same action, the dual feedback to your brain helps it interpret the data more accurately.

Here's another example. Try standing on one foot. At first, keep the foot in the air from touching anything else. Depending on your balance, standing on one foot may be hard or easy. Now try touching the foot in the air to the grounded leg. You may notice your balance suddenly gets better, or you can hold the pose for longer. You now have the feedback from both of your legs rather than just one. Try this out in different situations and see if you can feel your body reacting to the feedback of two limbs rather than one.

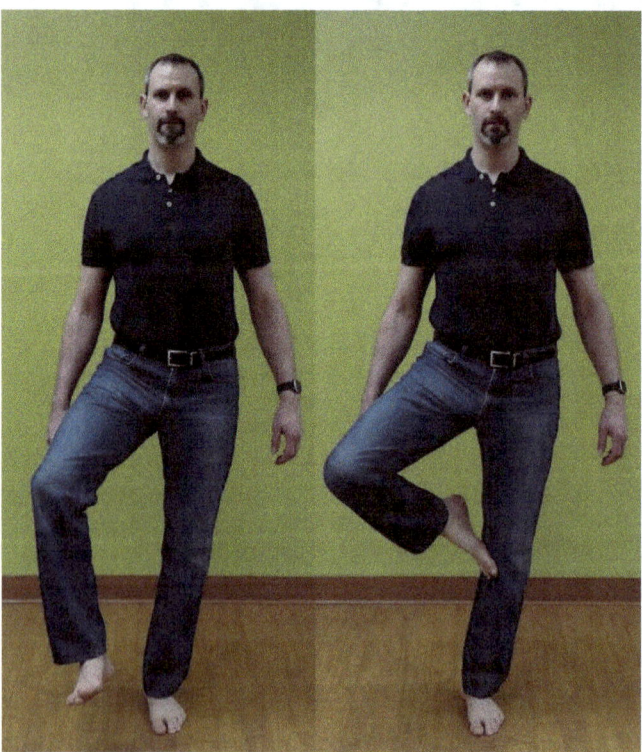

Figure 71: Standing on one foot without and with completing a circle. It takes less effort to balance with a complete circle.

A harder example than above, mainly because not a lot of people can do them, is pull-ups. If you can do one, try doing a pull-up with your feet separate, then a pull-up with your feet touching. You may find the second way is easier.

It's a simple idea that it is easier to do something if your muscles are acting together rather than opposing each other. This seems self-evident, but you would be surprised how often you let your muscles work against each other rather than with each other. Pay attention to your body and see if you can recognize times when you can be more efficient!

The Barrel

Moving from the idea of making a circle, here's another concept I greatly enjoy, and teach to all my martial arts students. It's not something innately part of a martial arts discipline, but it helps the application. It also helps in everyday life. This concept is the "barrel." To see how this works, put your arms out in front of you, palms facing toward you, one hand behind the other, as if you're holding a giant barrel. You don't want the barrel to fall, so you have to keep up tension while you hold it.

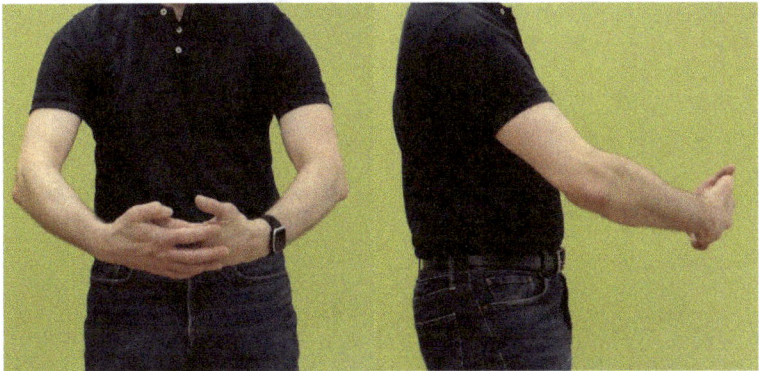

Figure 72: The "barrel." Hold your arms as if you are supporting a heavy pot or vase.

Ideally, you want to make the circle of your arms the same strength in every part. So, press out with your hands, your arms, your shoulders, and your back. You can test if your barrel is strong with somebody else's help. Have them randomly press on any part of the circle, and see if it collapses in. For a harder test, have them push against two opposing sides of your barrel, and see if it collapses. Often this will be at your elbows, or between your hands, or in the center of your back. Remember, joints are your weak points!

Why is the barrel important? This concept allows you to create a circle with your arms where force applied to them is deflected to the side. This means it's very hard to collapse. So what? Because you can use your arms when they are in "barrel form" to help you deflect incoming force. You can even keep the barrel going with only one hand. Go back to the example I showed you. Make a barrel out of your arms, then raise one hand higher and let the other one sink lower. You still have a barrel except your hands aren't actually touching. It's not as strong (because you're not completing a circle), but that doesn't always matter.

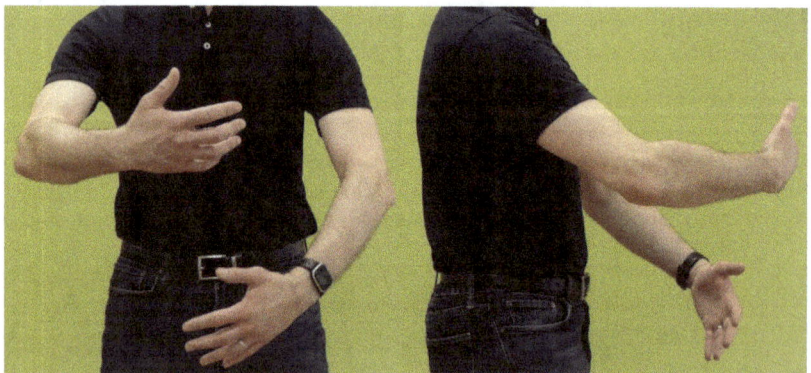

Figure 73: A separated barrel. There is less strength in this one, but more mobility.

Okay, here's a practical example. Find one of those big heavy metal doors with the press bar across them. Make a barrel with your dominant arm (or both together if you really want), then walk into the door (preferably on the bar section). Remember the theory! You never want your arm to collapse. In "barrel," your arm can take the load of your entire body walking into the door, pressing the release bar, and opening the door without collapsing. You can keep walking through the door with less reduction in your speed while doing so.

> You can use a regular wood door in your house, so you don't have to exert yourself pushing a release bar.

What if you're holding a heavy bag of groceries? Make a barrel with one arm to cradle the groceries against your side, or to hold them up by the handle. This is the same idea as someone cradling a baby against their hip.

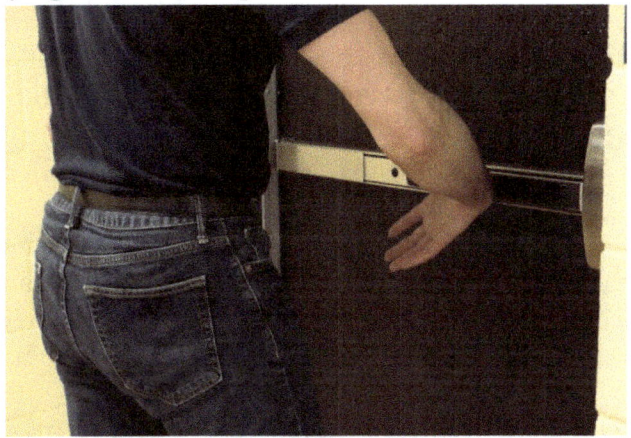

Figure 74: Using the barrel to open a door.

Don't want to touch a greasy banister in a public place? Try making a barrel with one arm and pressing the back of your wrist or your elbow against the banister rather than holding it with your open hand.

You can get the same steadying feedback the banister is there for, but you don't have to touch it with a body part that is going to be touching (potentially) your mouth, nose, or eyes. Even though you aren't actively gripping the banister, you're still getting the kinesthetic feedback to tell you where you are in relation to it, and in relation to how the stairs slope downward. This isn't going to save you from tumbling down the stairs if you pitch forward (for that, keep reading!), but it's likely to steady your balance enough so you don't do so in the first place.

Here's an example of using the barrel with your legs. If you're on an unstable surface, like a moving vehicle or boat, try making a barrel with your lower half. It's the same idea, except your feet aren't going to be on top of each other, obviously. Instead, think about pressure through your knees. You want pressure down and around the outsides of your legs, so that your feet start to rest on the outside "ridge" edge.

You can feel this sort of stance is the same as making a barrel with your arms. You'll have to bend your knees when you do it, but then, you should never have your knees locked out anyway. You will resist motion sideways to your body. If that doesn't resist the motion in the correct direction, put one foot about two of your foot lengths in front of the other. Then press out with the front leg and back with the rear leg, sort of like what we did in the isometrics warm-up.

I described using the ridge edge in the section on "wobbling" and in the anatomy section. Yes, I'm finally getting to that explanation, but not quite all of it!

This has the effect of creating a barrel oriented front to rear of your body rather than side to side. Depending on the direction of the motion you're dealing with, this stance should enable you to stay much more balanced.

There are a bunch of different applications for the barrel, which is why I like teaching it. Play around with it, with both your arms and your legs, and see if it helps you out too.

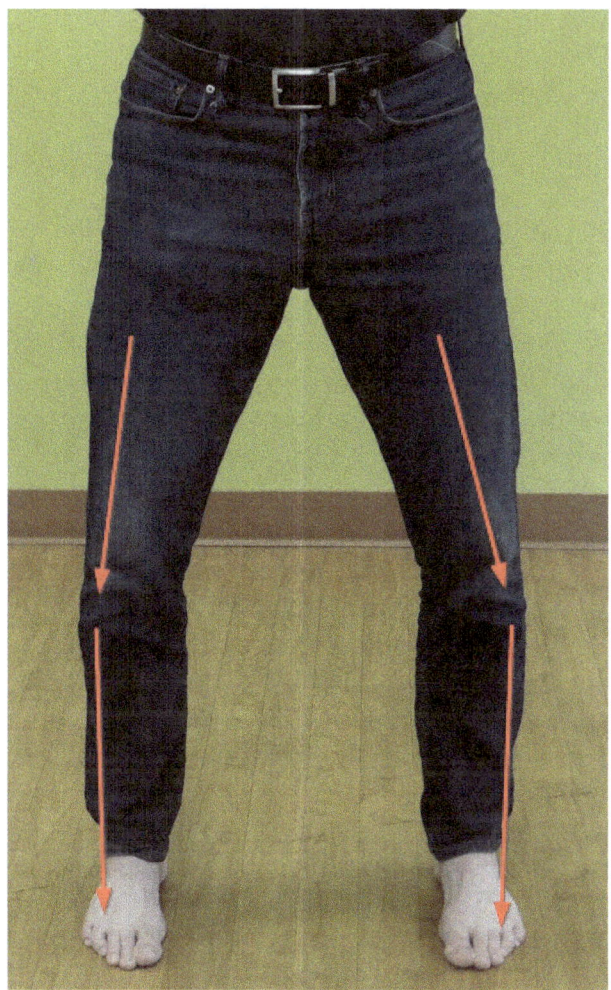

Figure 75: A barrel with the legs, oriented side to side. When attempting this you should feel pressure on the outside of your legs and feet.

The Core

As mentioned before, this could be a whole book on its own, but this is a great time to go into the muscles in your torso with more fine detail now you have anatomy, movement, and some concepts like the barrel under your belt.

First, we need some terms. I'm going to divide up your torso into two main areas. The first is the *core:* the squishy area with all the muscle that doesn't include your ribs. The second is the *mantle*: the part that houses the ribs and connects to the neck. If you move your torso around, you can feel a bit of difference between these two areas. The mantle is more rigid than the core, and the core is more maneuverable.

Let's start with the lower part of your torso. This part contains your center and connects directly to your legs. It has walls of muscle front and back, which keep all your insides in, but there is no bone protecting it. It's very good at absorbing blunt impacts. Not so much pokey ones (just ask the Pillsbury Doughboy). The only bone in it is the spine, which, coincidentally, also contains the lumbar area (that special human extra curve) that causes us so much pain. Why is this pain so common? My guess is, it has to do with most of us not keeping enough connection in the core to support the spine and thus keep it from twisting in ways that are painful (see toting around another person, above).

I talked about connection at the beginning of this book. Remember, you should not be completely relaxed, and not fully tense. Your muscles are engaged and ready. For your core, this means you are keeping your abs just tensed enough to make your belly feel "firm" instead of "squishy." This is the feeling on the inside wall of muscle—not the outside layer of fat we all have, by the way. You can do this no matter your body shape. Keeping connected like this has the added benefit of making you look trimmer! Activating your core pulls your belly in just a little, and also helps you stand straighter.

When your core is engaged, you're also protecting your spine from making sudden motions without the rest of your body. The "connected" muscle around it acts like a shock absorber, especially if you are dealing with heavy objects. Remember the exercises around your lower spine from the back anatomy section? It's easier to do these with engaged abs. Having control of these muscles will help you engage and connect all of the muscles in your core at once to protect your back from injury.

> Protecting your spine from injury is important! The more you are loose and in bad posture when you walk, the more of your weight you put directly on the bone and spinal discs.

Your core can also compress a lot. Imagine you have a stack of pancakes in your abs, and you squeeze down on them. If that comparison doesn't work for you, imagine you have a rubber ball and are squishing it between your ribs and your pelvis. If that doesn't work either, think about the feeling of zipping up tight pants. Feel free to come up with your own way to describe compressing your core. Whichever way you do it, it's a great way to solidify your core area and activate your pelvic floor.

This is not an easy concept, and especially not easy to remember to do all the time, but I promise it will help your posture and help prevent back injury. You might want to put this book down for a while and try it out for a few days. Set a timer and check every thirty seconds or so to see if you're keeping your core engaged. Go on. I'll still be here.

Waiting.

Once you feel like you've got the hang of compressing your core, it's time to bring in the transition space between your core and your mantle. What you want to do is compress your core down, but at the same time, stretch everything above the top of your core *up*. Try to feel a little space open between the top of your compressed core and the bottom of your ribs.

Let's move on to the other part of the torso, the mantle. This will probably be even less familiar to you than the core, as people can figure out how to compress their abs, but not their ribs. First, make sure you have good posture. It's hard to work with your mantle when you're slumped over. Head stretching up, shoulders back and down, hips tucked. Now feel the difference between your mantle, which is all the muscles and bone from your ribs to your neck, and the core, which is everything below that in your torso. Compress your core as above and make that little space under your ribs. Then try to turn just your mantle side to side, without moving your solid core. It's difficult, and you can't move a whole lot, but you can separate the two. You can even try to twist your core one way and your mantle the other way! Try not to waggle your shoulders around when you do this—they should be relaxed. The movement comes from your back muscles around your spine, not pulling your body around from the shoulders. Focus on feeling the twelve thoracic vertebrae connecting your ribs. These are the ones in your mantle.

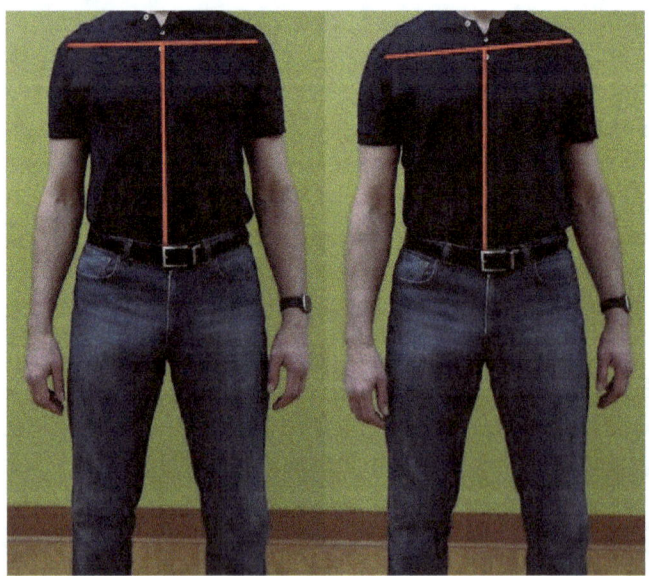

Figure 76: Torso straight (left) and with the mantle turned (right). Note the hips and belt are in the same position, so only the upper part of the torso is moving.

This can also take some time to feel. It's not something we do often and will likely be a new type of movement for you. Again, it's alright to put this book down for a while and spend a few days feeling out this type of motion.

...

Are you back, with new frontiers of movement opened up? Then, with good posture, a compressed core, and space between the core and ribs, try to compress your mantle down. It's sort of like you're lowering your ribcage down over that stack of pancakes, closing that open space between core and ribs. You can compress a good bit, making your whole torso very solid with mantle stacked on core. This is great to resist movement or support a heavy load, and it keeps your spine from twisting and injury. But, it does *keep* the spine from moving. You're not very mobile in this position, but you can support a lot of weight or resist an impact.

Now try the other way. Keep your core solid, but this time lift your mantle up, away from it. You're increasing that space between core and ribs, and you should feel the muscle there very expanded and solid. When you do this, you have greater flexibility and movement in your mantle, even though your core is less mobile. In this position, your lumbar vertebrae will be more protected from twisting, but you still have a good amount of flexibility to twist and reach with your mantle and arms.

What good is all this? An excellent question. Now I've made you wriggle around like you have a particularly itchy tag in your shirt, let's talk about the practical applications. I've mentioned a few already. Each of these options can protect your back from quick motion and injury in different situations.

Engaged core: this is good to do all the time, really. The more you do it, the stronger your abs will be. It's like always doing crunches or sit-ups! It will help your posture, your balance, and it will keep your belly looking trimmer. At least while you're standing, there's no real reason to lose this engagement and let your belly go "soft."

Compressed core: if you are picking up something heavy, this is a great way to protect your lower spine from accidental injury. It also moves your center slightly, and if you get really good at this, you can feel that it's lower and slightly forward, which gives you a better lifting base.

Compressed core, compressed mantle: now you're really not going anywhere. Need to resist a force or wind? Need to keep your back absolutely straight? Need to push up into an object or lift an object above your head? This solidifies your entire torso into basically a brick. Congrats, you're an immovable object.

Compressed core, raised mantle: this is both a solid position, and gives you room for manipulation. It's also the hardest to pull off, so don't worry if this takes you some time to feel. This is great if you need solidity in your legs, but also need to move your arms to reach or manipulate. You could use this while standing on a slippery or unstable surface, but need your hands free to do an action, for example.

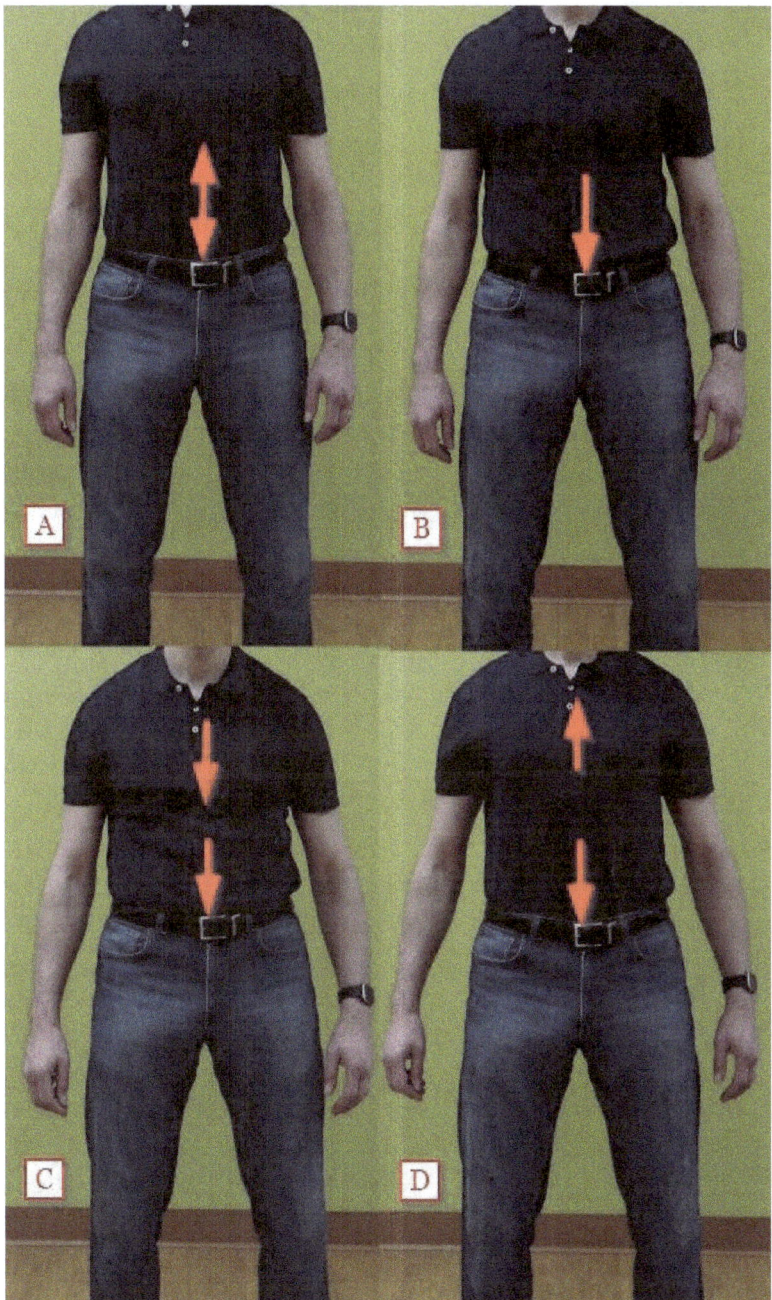

Figure 77: A: Engaged core, B: Compressed core, C: Compressed core, compressed mantle, D: compressed core, raised mantle. Note A and D look very similar from the outside.

Walking Through Doors

This is a natural extension of both the barrel and using your core. It's a cool efficiency of movement I employ nearly every day. How do you walk smoothly through a door rather than pausing to open and close it? This is going to be a little complicated to explain, but it's also almost the end of the book. You're an expert now!

You're going to be using all four of your extremities when you do this. Let's start with going through a door that opens away from you rather than toward you. First, make a barrel with the arm that's going to open the door and engage your core. Grip the door handle as you come close, but don't stop walking. Instead, keep your arm barreled and since you now walk with your center of mass moving forward in good posture, you can use your entire momentum to open the door as you walk through it. You may need to walk around the door slightly as it opens. But that's not all! Keep holding on to the handle, and once you're through the doorway, you can push on the handle, or move your hand to grab the edge of the door, while still keeping the barrel in your arm. Then shut the door behind you as you move through it. It's all one motion. You don't have to stop, push open the door, walk through the doorway, turn around, and push the door closed.

You may need to slow down for this one on the approach to the door. Make sure you can grip the handle and pull it toward you, rather than opening the door directly into your face (not a desired outcome).

Now let's try this with a door that swings toward you. This is more complex, because you have to pass the door from one hand to the other, but you've learned a lot about manipulation by now (see the dexterity section, below). Pull on the door and use the momentum of pulling the door toward you (covered in "muscles moving against each other") to step past it as it swings open. Next you will need to pass the door from the hand that opened it to your other hand, which should be behind you as you move through the doorway. Keep walking forward, and let your rear hand pull the door closed as you do so. Again, pretty much all one motion: open the door, pass through it, and close it behind you. If you don't want to close the door, you can instead let it continue to open behind you.

If you get good at this action, it makes moving through doorways very quick. Try it out with public bathroom stalls, because the doors are often spring-loaded, and close a lot more easily. But because you're in a confined space, you may need to use your newfound turning ability now you have excellent posture and are not slinging your center of mass around as you turn. There's plenty of space to turn between a stall door and a toilet, isn't there?

Walking Sideways

Now, I'm going to bring in an astonishing concept. Did you know your legs move sideways as well as forward and backward? This, *finally*, is what I wanted to talk about way back when I was explaining how your feet moved. But we needed all that explanation in the middle before I could explain it properly. So here it is.

What's the first step? Yes, that's right, good posture. If you're slumping for this one, it's not going to work as well. Stand up straight, then rather than taking a step forward, take a step to the side. Bend both knees a little bit and try to land just slightly on the outside ridge edges of your feet rather than flat. This is similar to rolling heel-toe, except you're going side-side. Lift up one foot just enough so it clears your other foot, move it across your standing leg, either in front or in back, and move your center of mass with it. If you stop at the midpoint of the step with your legs crossed, they will be crossed preferably above your knee height, both knees will be bent, and both feet will be planted on the outside ridge. Continue moving your center to the side, bring your other foot around, and plant it flat on the floor. Congratulations, you've just stepped sideways. Your next step will return to your feet being side by side as your foot that hasn't moved yet now follows through.

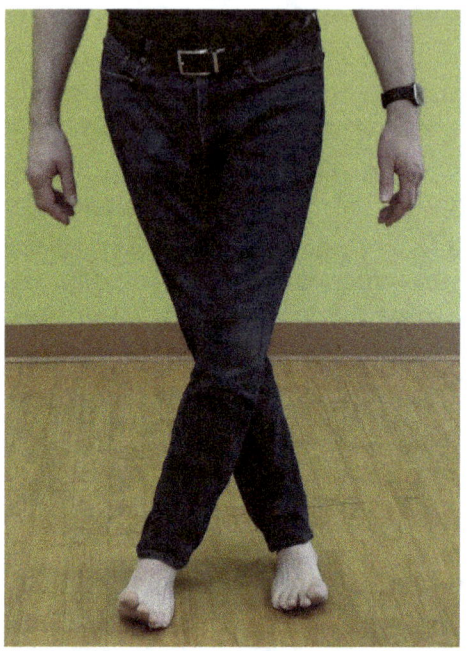

Figure 78: Stepping sideways on the ridge-edge of the feet.

Try this with your foot stepping across in *front* of your stationary leg and also *behind* your stationary leg, because you're going to use both ways. Attempt this sequence slowly to get used to stepping in a different direction than normal. Once you get some confidence in it, try stepping in front of your stationary foot on the first step. Then follow through so your feet are side by side again. On your next step, go behind your (new) stationary foot. Once you get good at it, it's almost as fast to walk sideways as it is to walk forward, especially if you're taking advantage of good posture to keep your center of mass where it's supposed to be.

But you're not going to be walking sideways all the time. Where is something like this useful? For me, the counter in my kitchen is laid out in a line—from the fridge to the sink to the stove. There are shelves above with cooking products. So, when I'm using the kitchen, rather than turn sideways and slumping along the counter until I get where I want to be, I simply step sideways. Say I'm washing a bowl in the sink. Finish washing, dry it off, step sideways to the correct cabinet, open it up (using your barrel, right?), bowl in, door closed, step sideways back to where I need to be.

Changing Directions with Your Arms

We'll change directions a bit both with this section and its outcome! Now you know how to control your core (because you did practice that bit above, right?) you can do amazing things by linking parts of your body together...more than they are already. Our muscles are extremely powerful, and if you compress and use connection—that feeling that isn't totally relaxed nor totally tense—you can line up your muscles and skeleton and use that to move more gracefully!

Remember the barrel, from a few sections back? We're going to need that again.

You can do all sorts of useful things with the barrel. Here's a few other things you can do with this concept.

Find that person who helped you test out your barrel before. This time, let's use your core as well! Compress your core and your mantle, like you've practiced. This makes your torso completely solid, and by using the barrel with your arms, they're now connected into your center too. Try to keep your barrel, and have your helper stand to one side and push on one of your arms, perpendicular to your body. They shouldn't be able to move you, because you're connected all the way from your arms to your legs. However, if you lighten your feet on the floor just a little (or if you're in socks on hardwood, or another low-friction surface), they will be able to push you around in a circle!

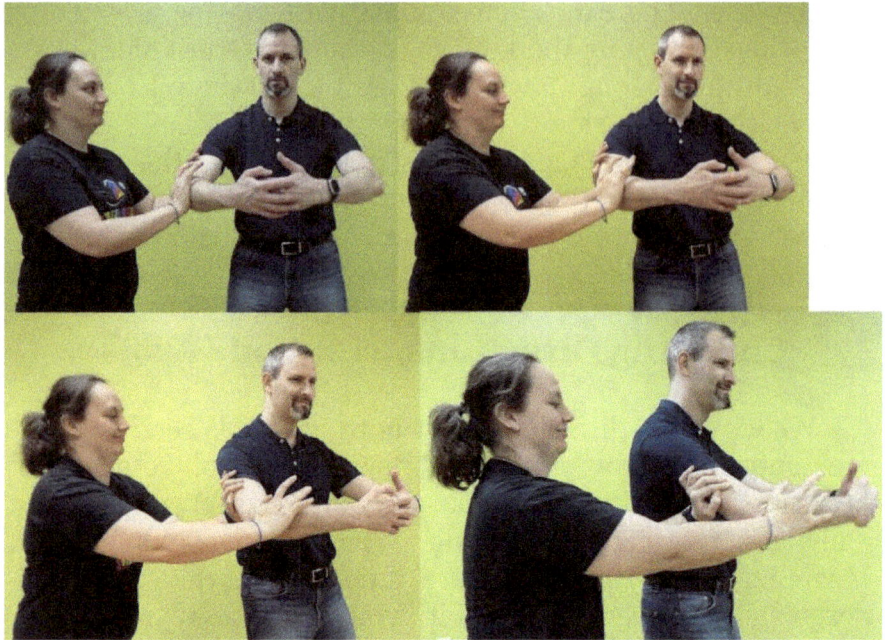

Figure 79: Your body is connected from head to toe in a good barrel position with an engaged core.

Aside from being a neat party trick, there are practical uses to this. If you relax the barrel on one arm, moving that arm can also make your whole body move. You can use this to your advantage if your core is connected to your legs and your mantle. Try relaxing one arm, moving it away from you quickly, then fixing your arm back in your barrel. Because you're arresting your momentum, and your body is connected to your arm, that energy has to go somewhere. The easiest way to dissipate it is for your body to "catch up" to your barreled arm, which means your body will move to one side. If you need to shift quickly to one side, for example while you're walking somewhere, this is a quick and easy way for your arms to help you change direction!

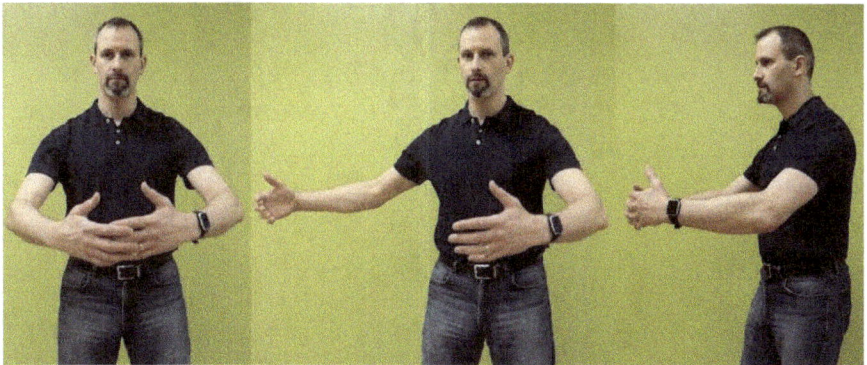

Figure 80: Relaxing one part of the barrel and then re-engaging can also turn your body!

If you practice this (like I do, because I'm strange), you can start to actually use other objects to redirect your motion. You can grab a doorway as you walk by it to turn into it quickly, push off or hold onto a banister to increase or decrease your speed, push away from counters or tables to start walking another direction, and so on. All this requires is some practice at the barrel position, along with control of your core and good posture. Once you figure out how to turn it on and off quickly, you can activate your barrel as you contact the other object and relax it as soon as you are past it. Keep practicing this! There are many more uses if you are able to control how your whole body moves at once.

You can also practice turning your torso to avoid objects. This will move your shoulders out of the way, reducing your outline and keeping your shoulder from ramming into a doorway, for example.

Dexterity, or How to Use Both Hands

In my late teens, I took up juggling, and practiced enough to get pretty decent at it, for example juggling four balls with a friend, and even managing to juggle five balls (for a very short period of time). Although I don't practice regularly anymore, I occasionally juggle for the fun of it. However, the reason I'm telling you this is that learning to juggle gave me a lot of benefit in the realm of dexterity. Being able to move three objects between two hands is great, and a lot of fun, but more important for everyday life is being able to move *one* object between *two* hands.

I'm not going to teach you how to juggle here (although I would recommend looking it up if you want to learn. There are a lot of great resources and it's very good exercise), but I am going to talk about the main benefits you get from thinking of objects as able to pass from one hand to another.

Find a smallish, round object that fits well in your hand and isn't going to break if you drop it on the floor. A tennis ball, golf ball, bean bag, baseball, apple, orange (if you don't mind bruised fruit), or something else. Hold it in your dominant hand, relaxed by your side, and have your other hand out in front, near your center. Now simply bring your dominant hand up and put the object into your other hand. Drop your dominant hand back down to your side. Then bring that hand up again and take the object from your non-dominant hand.

That's the basics of juggling! Try the same thing with your non-dominant hand holding the object by your side and bring it up to pass to your dominant hand in front of your body. Try this out for a while until it feels natural on both sides. This is one of those places where it's okay to put this book down and try this exercise over a few days.

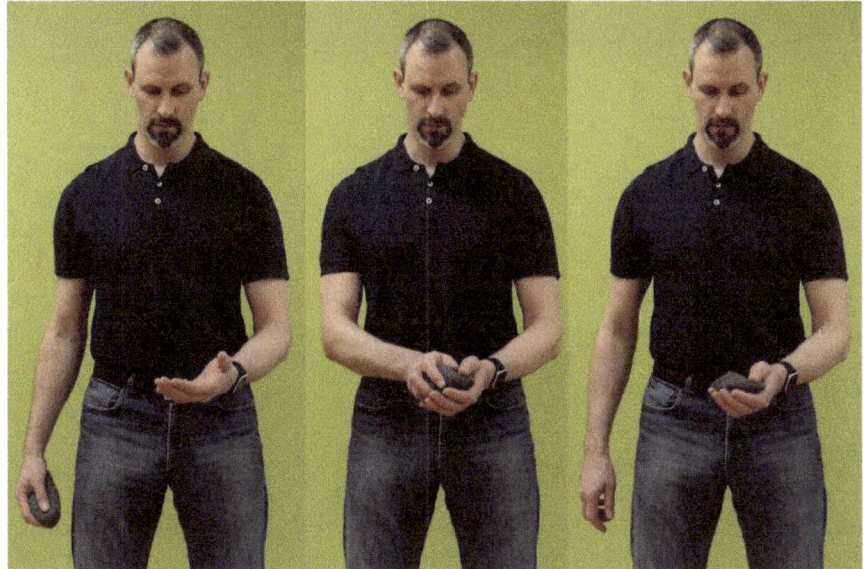

Figure 81: Pass an object to your other hand, then do the opposite and remove an object from your hand.

...

Back already?

If you have that part down, then try the next step. Start with both hands by your side, bring them both up, pass the object from one to another, and drop both back to your sides. Repeat, passing the other way. Practice this until it's smooth and natural. As you do, you might notice you're actually throwing the object a tiny distance between your hands as you pass it. If this happens, let it. Try to throw a slightly farther distance. You're making new connections in your brain of how to operate your body, learning where objects are and should be based on your body's movements (see "proprioception" in the section on how to pick things up). Eventually, you can even do this without looking at what you're passing, because your body is so used to doing it, your receiving hand knows exactly where the object should be.

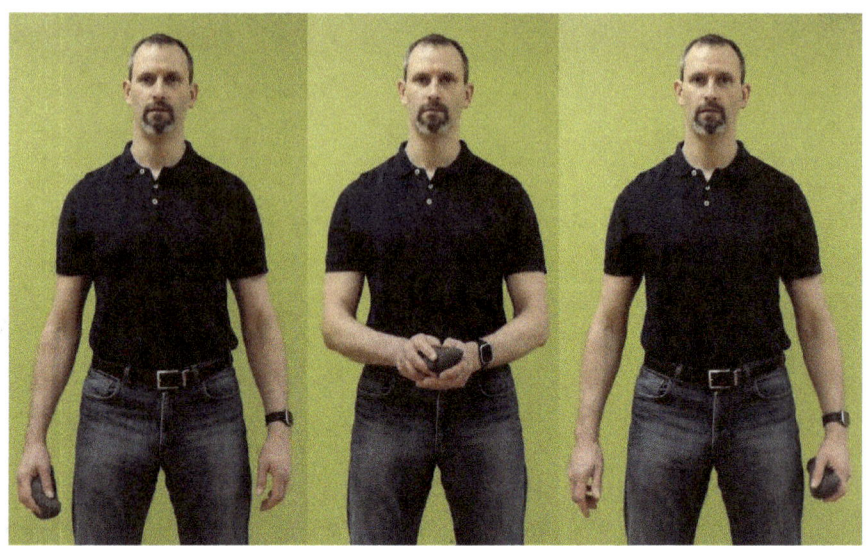

Figure 82: pass an object between your hands without looking at it. Then pass it back.

Even more than juggling, this is one of the most important dexterity skills you can have. Learning where an object is in relation to your body opens up that "field" of area in your mind, and now instead of limiting yourself to the items directly on you or in your body, you start to realize where objects are around six inches (fifteen centimeters) or so away around you. These aren't just things you're holding, but obstacles and other people, which keep you from running into them.

Keep practicing switching objects from hand to hand. Aside from posture (which you're still paying attention to, right? Remember to keep your head up and shoulders back and down), this is one of the most important concepts in this book. As you get better with moving

Always remember you have two hands (assuming you do)! If so, then don't let one hand dangle uselessly while you perform some action. How can it help? Creating a circle? Holding an object? Doing another action at the same time?

items around, you may find yourself naturally changing hands to use things, like switching your phone from one hand to the other to take out your keys, or passing a cup of water to your non-dominant hand to take something another person gives you.

Your hands aren't the only option, either! Remember the discussion about how many joints you can use to hold objects? Maybe you've got a water bottle in your dominant hand. Except your phone rings. So you pass the water to your non-dominant hand, and answer your phone. But then you need to get into your home, so pass the water bottle to your elbow and cradle it against your side while you pass the phone to the other hand to keep talking. You open the door and bump into a side table, knocking a vase off, so you can twist the keys around in that hand to put a finger through a keyring and use your hand to catch the vase, all while still talking on the phone and carrying your water. It sounds like an action comedy with Jackie Chan, but you can do this too! Guess what actor *really* knows how to operate his body?

As you are twirling three or four objects between your hands, you're going to drop one now and then. Fortunately, working on the ability to pass an object from one hand to another also boosts your reaction speed. That's the time it takes for your brain to process an event has happened and decide to do something about it.

Increased reaction speed is an amazing boon. You'll find yourself doing things you didn't think were possible, like dropping an object, then catching it with the same hand before it hits the ground. I'll often grab for an object I drop even before I know I'm doing it. That's because grasping is an innate action for us humans, and boosting your reaction time by passing objects back and forth puts grabbing and using objects into muscle memory, which means your brain doesn't have to include you in the decision to act. It just does. This is the basis of training in martial arts, where experienced practitioners might look like they're moving almost before they need to block or strike.

I made a presentation on martial arts, back in my first days of working at a large corporation, and talked about how reaction time could help you catch a pen or bottle of water that fell off your desk. I demonstrated in the presentation, with no desk, pen or water bottle, just moving my hand in the air, and for some reason got a bunch of "Ooohs" from the audience. A fast reaction time is impressive to other people, no matter what you're doing!

How Not to Hurt Things

If you are moving efficiently and quickly, or moving large objects around, there is more opportunity to hurt yourself. Now you are getting adept at operating your body, let's look at some ways to protect yourself in everyday life. This will use all three sections of your body: your legs, arms, and core.

How Not to Hurt Your Neck

NOTE: Take this section with a generous portion of the I Am Not a Doctor I mentioned in the forward. These are techniques that I've found work for me. However, doing too many of these neck exercises with an injury may cause more injury if you're not careful. So be gentle while you figure out How to Operate Your Body!

Have you turned your neck wrong and then not been able to move your head for a couple days? Your neck is almost comically easy to misalign and not that easy to put back into place. It's a common problem not just for humans, but for anything that has a neck. It's a weak and exposed area, but it makes up for that weakness in the ability to swivel and give the owner a full range of motion. These seven vertebrae (in almost all mammals) give a good range of ability to twist left and right, and curve up and down. In addition, you can press forward and back a little and even tilt left and right. These are the four main degrees of freedom.

In general, I've noticed most of my neck pain or seizing up happens when I move my neck "strangely" in more than one of these degrees of freedom. For example, just prior to writing this, I managed to cramp my neck while washing my hair in the shower (because I'm old). But breaking this down, I accidentally pressed too hard at the wrong angle. I activated two degrees of freedom at once: moving backward and tilting backward at the same time. You might also sneeze while turning your head (moving forward and twisting left or right) or sleep wrong (usually twisting and tilting backward or forward). I've even almost choked before by swallowing just as I was twisting my head to the side. The neck is full of (stupid) dangers.

> The neck is a very large, multifaceted joint, and joints are weak spots! The muscle in your neck is also not as tight to the bone as in your knees or elbows because your neck moves in more directions, so it's not as protective.

Because those seven vertebrae are all lined up in a column around your spinal cord, they have freedom to twist and move. Their downfall is when they press against each other at an angle by moving in two directions at once. This cramps up that vertical column, makes your muscles scream in agony, and now you can't turn your neck for three days.

Can I help you to never do this again? Probably not (see above where I took a shower "wrong"). But now you are at least more aware of the problem areas in moving your neck. So the next time you're craning your neck, or trying to tilt to the side while craning forward, be careful in your motion so you don't get a pain in the neck!

If I can't keep you from ever doing this, I should at least give you some tips to help out when you invariably hurt your neck. First, try gently stretching your neck in all four degrees of freedom. Depending on what you hurt, some directions will be more uncomfortable than others. This is good information to have. It tells you where the problem is. *Gently* stretch your neck out in the direction that hurts. This, again, is the difference between "uncomfortable" and "pain" I talked about at the beginning of the book. You can change the feeling from "pain" if you move your neck too fast while it's injured, to "uncomfortable" by gently approaching the pain point. Press a little farther into the "pain" zone as you stretch your neck, and it may help to reduce the time it takes for the muscle pain to go away.

If you get some experience at this (I'm sorry, because this means you've hurt your neck multiple times like I have), you can start to feel the two directions in which the muscles around your neck are inflamed, thus causing pain. It may be even more effective to move your neck *gently* in the two directions you originally injured it. It's often best to go in one of the directions, then start moving your neck slowly in the second direction to figure out where the injury is. For example, you might tilt your neck back, and then slowly tilt left or right, if that's where your discomfort is.

This is also a good time to do the muscle massages I showed in the anatomy section on the neck: rubbing up the trapezius toward the neck, and digging fingers into the trapezius. I've found if I can loosen the area up enough, and then gently move my neck around, finding the injured area, I can sometimes "pop" my neck back to where it's supposed to go, realigning the vertebrae. If these simple exercises don't work, or make things worse, definitely see someone in the medical profession for another opinion.

How Not to Hurt Your Back

This one is a little easier to prepare for than the neck, because there is so much muscle and structure around your back. This depends highly on the section about the core, in Body Mechanics. If you haven't read that yet, do it now.

Hopefully you've at least tried out engaging and compressing your core, and raising and compressing your mantle. Even if you haven't been able to feel out the muscles, just being aware of those positions will help keep you from injuring your back.

Like the neck, if you start twisting your back in two directions at once, that's when you're most likely to injure it. Added to that, your back is where all that load goes when you lift something, so if you've raised a heavy object off to one side or far away from your center, there's an increased likelihood you messed up your back. I did this recently shoveling mulch. I reached just a little too far and pried up on the shovel when it was pointing away from my body. I felt the "pop" in my back as something moved out of place. As above, moving slowly and planning where you want to go will save you a lot of neck and back ache!

As before, I want to include a section on what to do when you invariably *do* mess up your back. Just like with your neck, it's probably still going to happen. The best way to reduce the time your body is injured is, again, to stretch. Your back has the same mobility as your neck, to a lesser extent, and you can feel out the strain in the same way. If it's in your lumbar area (which it's likely to be) then doing the exercises I outlined in the part on isolating the deep back muscles can help. Isolating individual vertebrae can help you feel out where the injury occurred and what muscles need to relax or move.

Secondly, there are some other stretches, some of which were covered above. I'll go over the back hanging stretch again here in brief (now you know more about your core). To do this, set your legs wide and bend your knees just slightly. Then you can bend forward and try to let your hands touch your toes. If they can do that, start relaxing until your entire upper body weight is hanging from your spine. This is one case where you want to relax completely! Let your core and mantle go soft so gravity stretches them out. It may help to twist or tilt your spine from side to side to open it up. Stay in this state as long as you like, slowly releasing muscles across your back and lengthening your stretch. If your hands touch the floor, you can cross your arms to give you some more room. As you stay in this position, you'll find more places to relax and open up your spine. If you have existing back problems, you might want to get the advice of your doctor before doing this stretch. When you finish, come up *slowly*! Re-engage all the muscles and pull up to standing position gradually, so all the blood doesn't rush from your head.

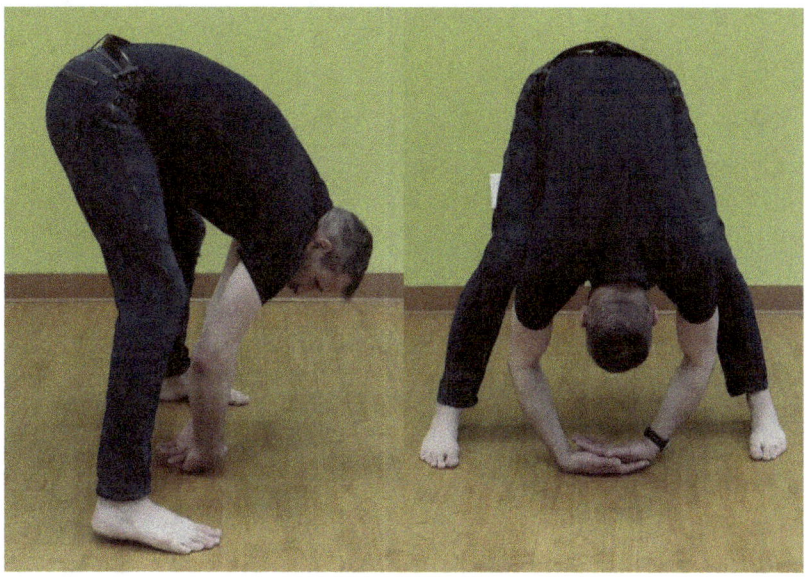

Figure 83: Stretching out the back (this is the same as Figure 23).

To save a little bit of time and space, since this is easily accessed information, I'll also give you a sequence of three yoga stretches I've found to target the lumbar area in particular and help reduce injury there. You can look up the exact methods and positions for: Downward Facing Dog, Cobra and Child's Pose. Following the instructions for these poses correctly plays a big part in helping your back, so here are a few tips. For Downward Facing Dog, make sure to press your hips backward in the pose. This will open up your lower back. Your heels may not touch the floor, and that's okay. For Cobra, make sure to slowly relax your lower back to get a really good stretch. Experiment with looking left and right over your shoulders. If Cobra feels like too much for you, try Sphinx Pose as an alternative. For Child's Pose, you also want to push your hips back, and you can also try looking left, right and center in the pose, because moving your neck may help to open up your lower spine as well.

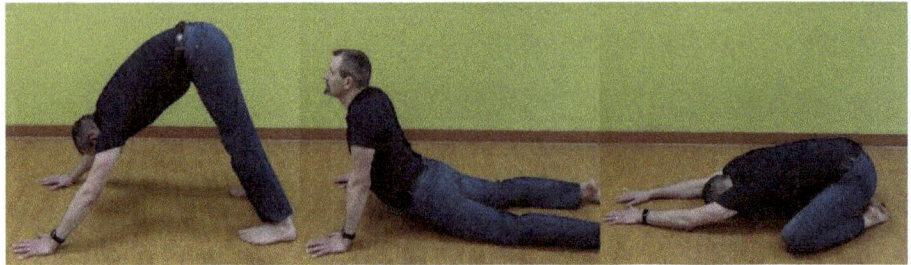

Figure 84: Downward Facing Dog (left), Cobra (middle), and Child's Pose (right).

I tend to go through this sequence: Forward Fold (the back hang from above), Downward Facing Dog, Cobra, Child's Pose, back to Cobra, back to Down Dog, and repeat these three as needed. Once you get used to them, vary the sequence up to see what helps you more. I've heard an audible *crack* before when doing these as my vertebrae go back into alignment. Always feel out what you're doing. Bending side to side or pressing slightly down or up in these poses can open up your spine in different ways. Just be careful and go slow. You're adjusting your spine alignment while doing this, and it's possible to do it wrong and make the injury worse if you go too fast!

How Not to Hurt Yourself Falling

This is one of the more complex sections of the book, and as such, I've saved it for last.

At some point it will happen. You, as a clumsy bipedal human, will trip, or overbalance, or be pushed over by someone or something. At this point, gravity takes over as you see the floor looming up toward you.

But all is not lost! Even if you trip over the cat in the dark, there are ways to keep from faceplanting. We're going to go over some of those here, using your legs, arms, and core.

You can get used to falling by simply doing so and figure out how not to land on bones or twist limbs under you.

Breaking this down to even simpler exercises can make you more comfortable with which parts of your body interface better with hard horizontal objects.

It's easiest to try this out on carpet or a foam mat (if you have one handy). We'll start from a prone position and work up to what happens when you come from a vertical position. First, lie down on the floor. If that's not something you do often, this is a great time to practice the basics of falling! Try to start by bending your knees rather than bending from your waist. Remember to fight off that robot menace! It's harder to lean over from your waist, then bend your knees,

We'll go through some more intensive body movements in this section. They're worthwhile to try out, but this is the one place I'll say it's okay not to do the exercise if you feel uncomfortable. If you do want to try them out, remember to go slow!

than it is to bend the knees first, then bend at the waist as needed to get your hands on the floor. Try reaching back with one or both hands as you bend your knees and waist so they are behind you. This makes it easier to plant your butt on the floor. Once that part of your anatomy is down, you can use its handy cushion for stability while you straighten your legs and upper body to lie prone.

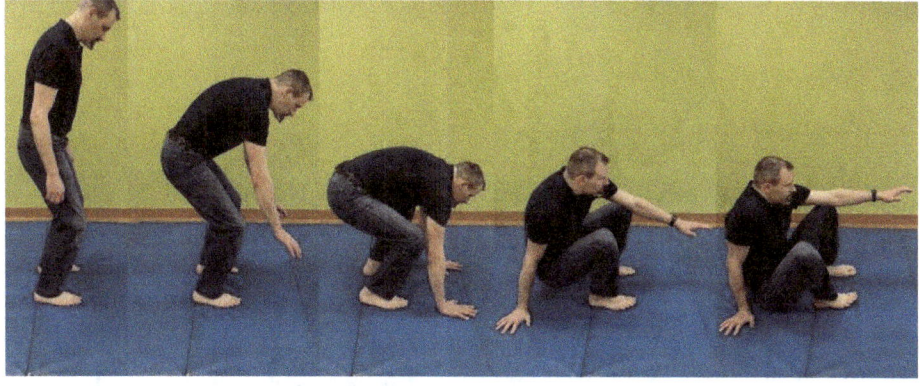

Figure 85: Getting down to sitting on the floor from standing. Start by bending your knees.

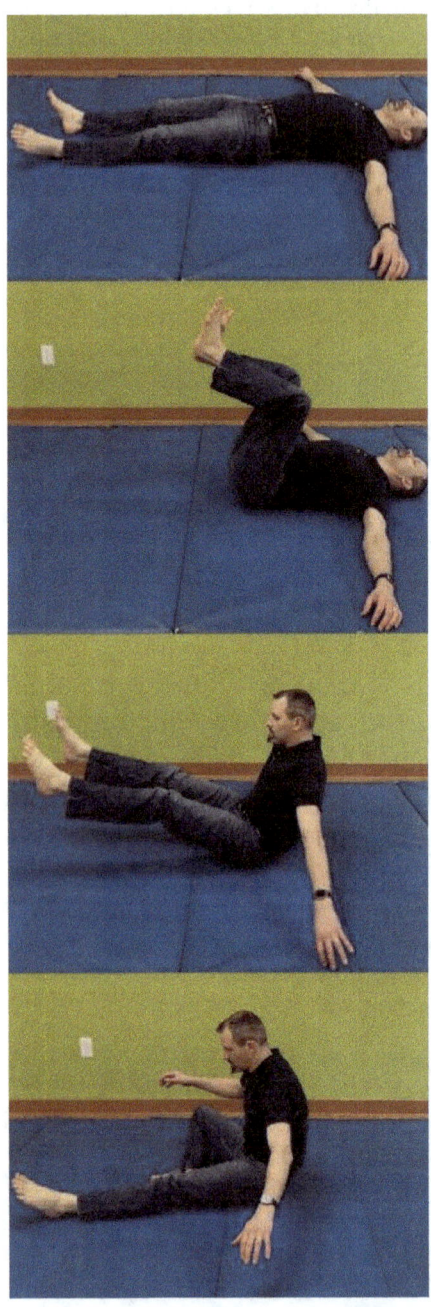

Figure 86: Rolling from prone to sitting.

You did it! Now what?

Learning how to move while prone is actually quite important. While you're lying on your back on the floor (still reading this book, I assume), bring your knees up, engage your core, and extend your legs with some force to rock forward. If you want to go more left, keep your left leg extended and tuck your right leg into it, and vice versa for the other side. With a little practice, you should be able to end in a sitting position, one leg extended.

Now you know how to sit up, we can do the reverse. From a sitting position, you want to rock backward, still with a connected core, so that your legs come up above you. There are two important things to be aware of while rolling! First, *keep your chin tucked* toward your chest so you don't hit your head on the floor. Second, *don't reach back with your elbows.* Doing so will engage the bony end of your elbow into the hard horizontal surface, and it will not be *humerus*. Or rather, that's what will hurt. If you need somewhere to put your hands, leave them out in front of you, reaching up.

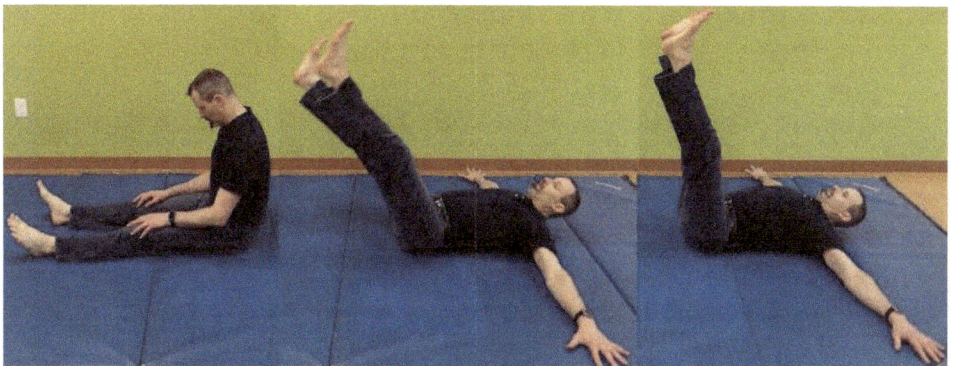

Figure 87: When rolling back, make sure to tuck your chin and don't bump your elbows!

Try to connect these two motions. You can make them feed off each other, so you rock forward, push away and rock back, and repeat. For an extra flair, try tucking your right leg into the left when your legs come up in the air, then roll slightly to the left when you go forward. The next time, tuck the other foot and roll to the right, so your shape is like a "V."

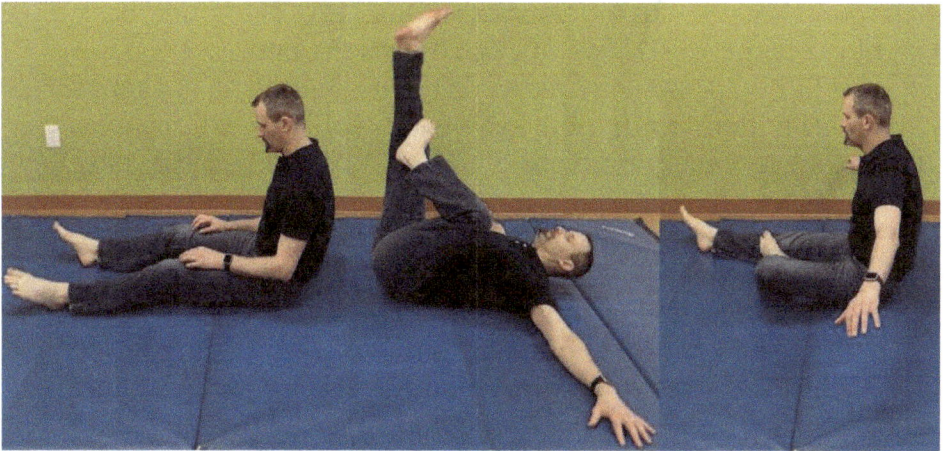

Figure 88: Rolling back and forward with one leg tucked. You can go to the side of the extended leg to make a "V" from your original location.

Once you have the hang of rolling, you can try stopping on your back, rather than stopping when your feet touch the ground. The most important part of this is *don't reach back with your elbows or your head*! Remember how I said to keep your arms in the air in front of you? Now you can start to use your arms. First check that you have your armspan length free around you. Then, as you rock back, *keep your arms straight* and try to place the palms of both (straight) arms on the floor directly out to either side. This will make it harder to roll forward again, but that's alright! You're stopping your motion. As you get used to rolling backward and stopping, you can use more force and slap the floor with your palms. Still keep your arms straight, though, and *don't bend your elbows*! Seriously, it will hurt if you do. Try to slap at exactly the same time as your back (with your chin tucked forward) also hits the ground. Making your hands, arms, and back all contact the floor at the same time dissipates the energy across a larger surface so you feel less impact. See the rightmost picture in Figure 87 for an example of what this looks like.

And I've already taught you most of what you need to know, at least for falling backward! How does rolling around on the floor translate to falling? The front/back rolling is the key. If you fall backward, the best case to stop your fall with the least injury is to roll onto your back and slap the floor with both palms, just like when rolling. Getting to that part from a vertical position is the next challenge.

Again, try a soft carpet, or a futon, or mat, or any other soft surface that's low to the ground. Start with the back roll from above, but this time instead of starting from sitting, start from a crouch. From standing, do a good squat (your balance over your heels) and then finish planting your butt on the floor and roll backward as above. Slap your hands (not your elbows) to arrest your motion.

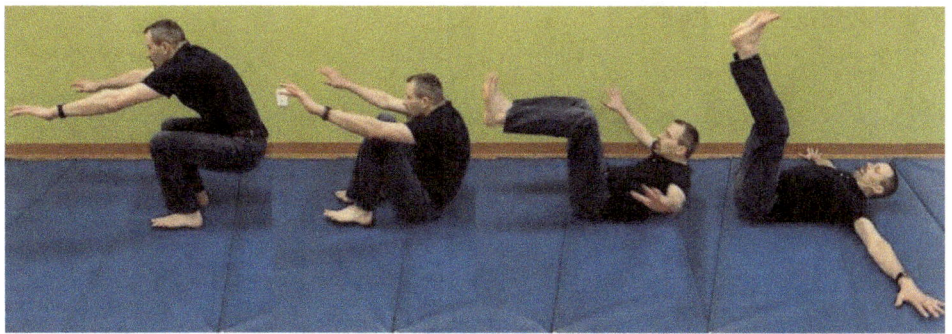

Figure 89: Controlled falling from a squat position.

From this point, it's up to you! Keep practicing your roll and getting into it from a squat. Remember to put your butt on the floor first, tuck your chin, and don't land with your elbows. As you get more comfortable, you can raise your squat and start the fall from a higher position. Eventually, you should be able to "fall" backward, bend your knees and roll to a stop safely on the ground.

And that's how not to hurt yourself falling backward. But what if fate is not kind and pushes you a different way?

Falling to your side is almost exactly the same as falling on your back. Remember the V-rolls? Those will be a big help here. Keep practicing them. If you start to fall to the side, again, bend your knees and lead with your butt. There's a reason we humans have a nice cushion there. The gluteus muscle and your upper thighs usually have a comfortable amount of fat, which helps to soften a landing and dissipate energy. So when falling to the side (see Figure 90), bend the knee on that side more than the other and as your butt touches the ground, tuck it into your other leg. Then do your V-roll. Even if you are turned and roll along your side instead of your back, it's a much softer landing. And since you are going down closer to one arm than the other, remember to stick both of them out in front of you! *Don't reach back with your elbows!* This is one of the most common ways to break a wrist. Our arms are really not cut out for resisting our entire body weight in a shock. Our butts and back, however, are big enough to spread out the energy.

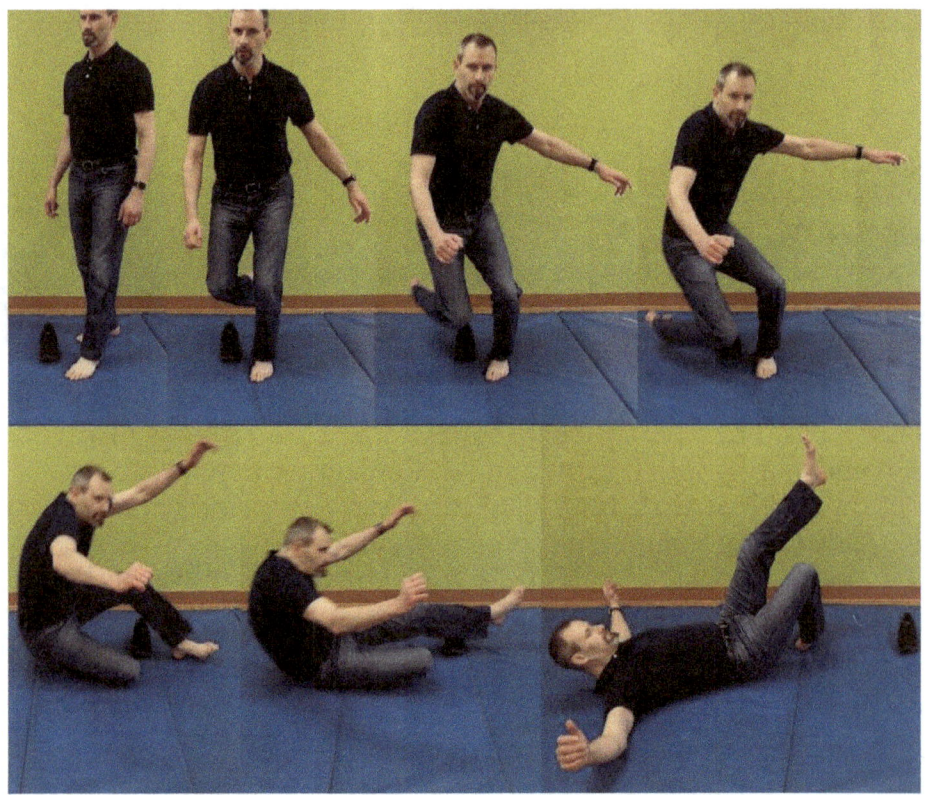

Figure 90: A sequence of how to fall to the side.

Now the hardest one. What if you trip over that cat and fall forward?

First, watch out for the danger points. These are your face, your shoulders, your wrists, your elbows, and your knees. Landing directly on any of these surfaces can cause breakage, or at least very least bruising and rashes. Just like above, you want to avoid hard contact with the ground, but since our knees don't bend forward, it's harder to control your fall because you can't sit your butt on the ground. We'll go in order of best case to worst.

> Remember: joints are weak points. Protect them!

Best case: if you have some warning, or some room, turn sideways as you fall. This might be easy to do if you've tripped and one foot is up anyway. Tuck it in, bend your knees, keep your arms away from the floor, and twist this into a side roll, just like we covered above. Watch your head on nearby objects (if at all possible). You may find you're rolling more across your back rather than up it, but that's fine. Curl up in a ball and tuck your chin to your chest as you fall. You don't want any bones or joints to hit any hard surfaces.

Next best case: you can't fully turn into a side roll, but you can turn. You can still prevent a lot of impact this way. First, bend your knees! Aim for the side of your thigh when you fall (NOT the pelvic bone). You can fall along your side, which is not ideal, but you can still spread the impact out along your core and ribs, up to your shoulder. Don't reach for the floor with a hand! Just don't do it. Keep the hand on your falling side out in front of you (parallel to the floor) and if you time it right, you can still slap your hand down to help disperse the impact even more.

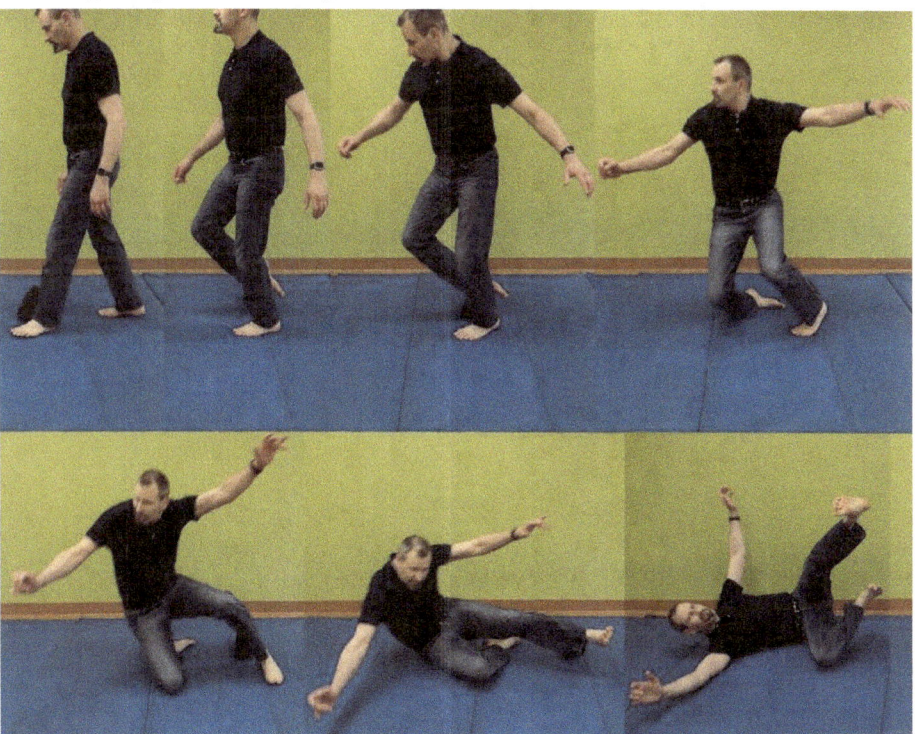

Figure 91: Turning from a front fall to landing on your side.

Worst case: you're falling straight forward. There's no time or space to turn. In this case, it's best to relax. Bend your knees. Crumple to the floor. There are not really any good surfaces to roll on, but you can tuck everything in and maybe land on your side. Don't reach for the floor with your hands! You do want to protect your face, however, and you can try to lay your entire forearm out to catch your fall. It's not ideal, but it will still stop you and disperse some of the impact, though you're likely to have bruises and rashes on your arms, especially if you fall on a hard surface like concrete. The more you can simply drop with knees bent, rather than tipping over, the better. But if you've moving fast and trip, you might be going straight down. Try to relax and bend your knees as much as possible, but this is where you may need to use your arms to protect your face. Turn your face to the side as well, to prevent falling straight onto your nose.

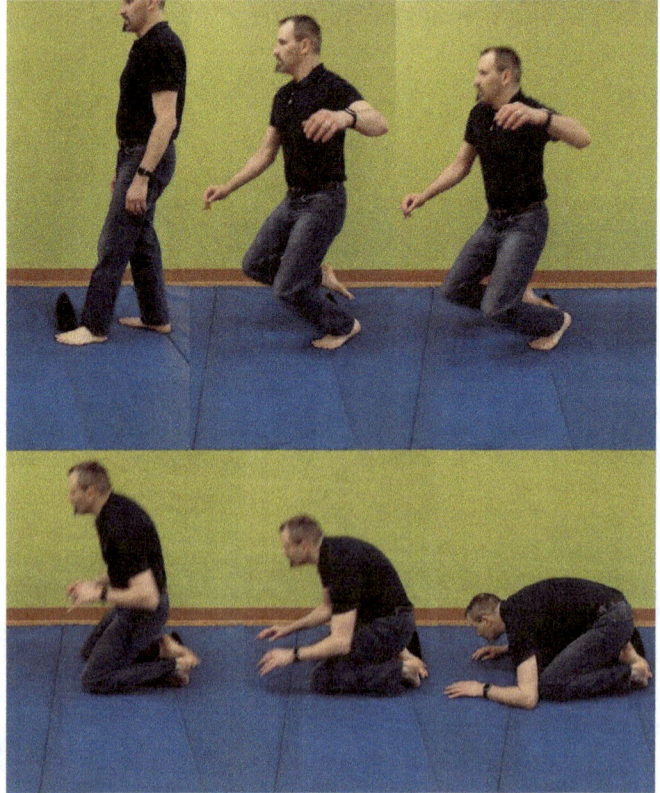

Figure 92: With nowhere to fall, it's best to collapse to your knees. You may need to use the flat of your forearms to keep from hitting your face.

There is one more way to stop a forward fall, but it's scarier to most people than just falling down, even though it's pretty easy to do and avoids more injury. You can roll forward, especially if you have momentum. As you're falling, bend your knees, tuck your chin, turn your head, and whichever way you naturally turn your head, aim the back of the *opposite* shoulder toward the floor. Your momentum will roll you over your shoulder and down your back, and you'll end up in that sitting "V' position!

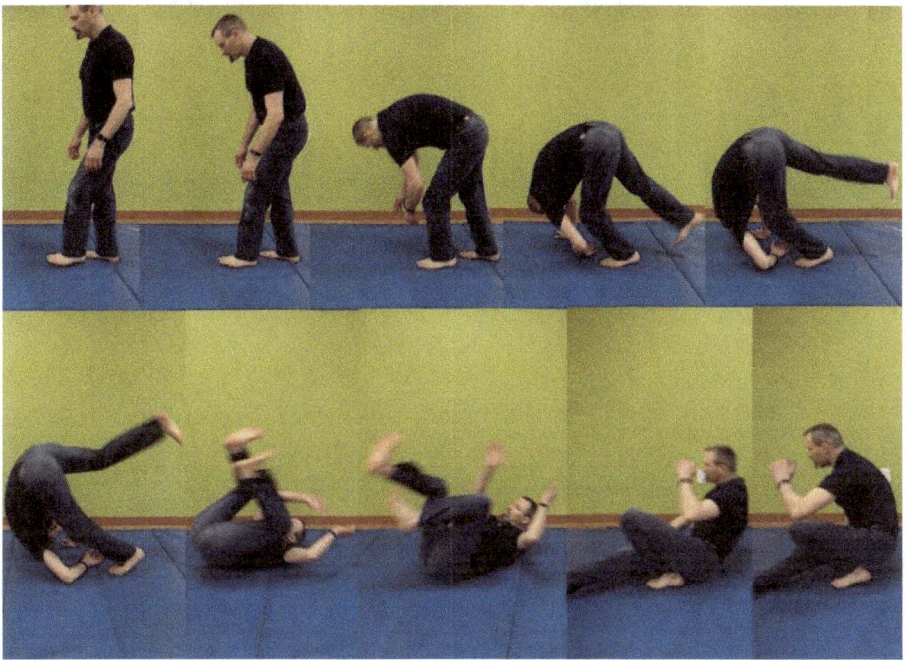

Figure 93: A full roll from standing. This can be used to avoid falling on your face, with practice.

This is, of course, easier said than done, but you can practice a simple version so you're more ready if you do fall. Get back to your soft rug, mat, or futon, and squat. Turn your head and tuck your chin, and again, point the *opposite* shoulder toward the floor. Try not to bang your knees on the floor when you do this. If you go slow, you may end up rolling across your back, rather than straight down. As long as what you do doesn't cause impact to bones and joints, it's a better way to fall than flat on your face!

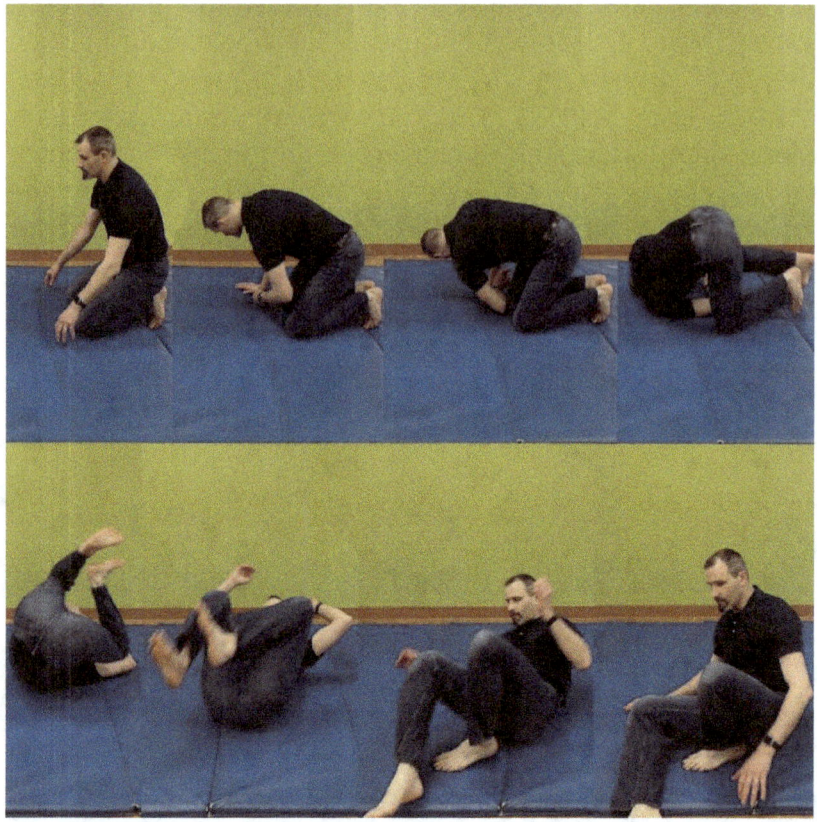

Figure 94: Learning a simple roll is a good way to practice keeping your joints safe!

You can also take a lesson from these falling and rolling exercises above even while you're standing. If you bump into someone or something (say, a door frame), thinking about how you roll on the floor when falling is the same concept as if you impact a hard surface when upright. Make sure not to clash any of your bones or joints against that other object. Instead, roll on your upper arm and back of your shoulder if possible. You can also use your barrel in this instance. Making a firm connection between your arm and body will let you roll around an obstacle, and rather than the impact going directly into your body, it's redirected to the side. This will reduce any bruising or impact you might suffer.

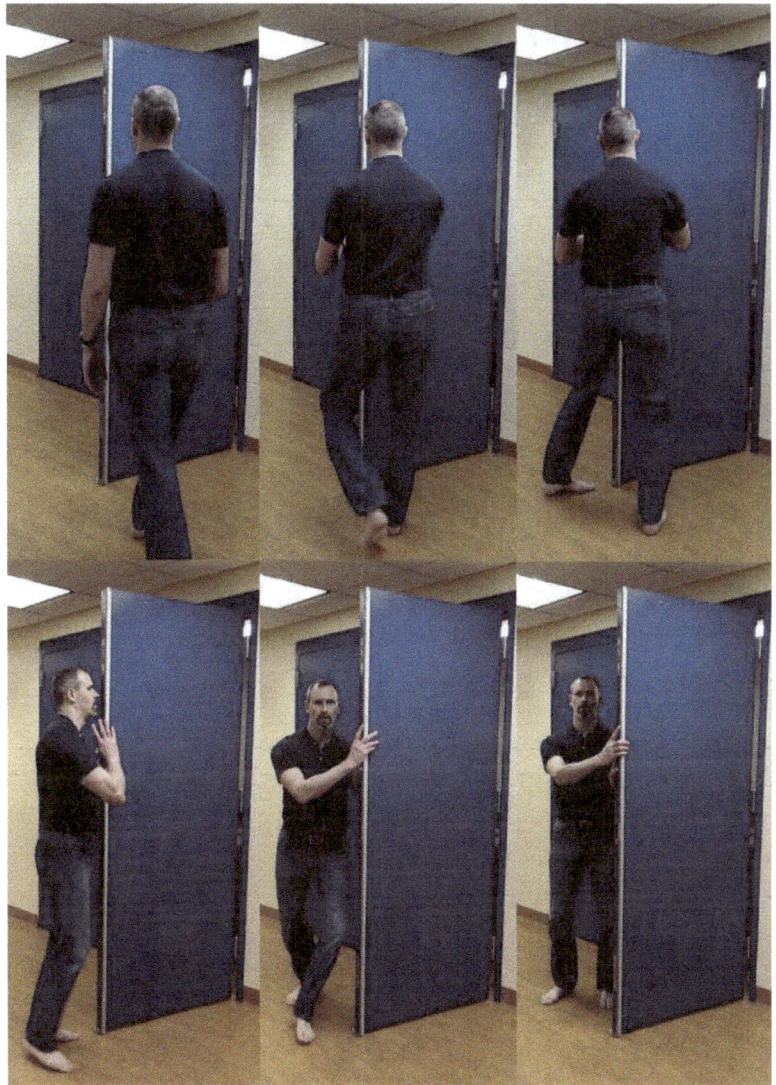

Figure 95: Rolling vertically around an obstacle.

There are a lot of *very* complicated actions in this section, and I can only describe so much in text. Just like in the rest of the book, this is a great place to practice a little here and a little there, working up to a roll or a fall. I'll also have some further actions in the wrap-up at the end of the book if you're interested in learning these techniques more in-depth or with a teacher.

The Four Quadrants of the Body

Let's bring together everything and look at the body as a whole. You're basically a torso with four appendages and a head attached. The torso and core provide stability and connection through the parts of the body, with the real foundation of the body being the spine. The lower limbs are big and powerful, with muscles that can support the weight of the body for long periods of time. The upper limbs are dexterous and nimble, able to manipulate one object with extreme precision, or multiple objects with skill, however they aren't as good at supporting body weight. Finally, there's a sensory and planning center placed on top, to help direct and coordinate all the parts.

The center of a standard human body is right below and behind the bellybutton. Being aware of this place will enable a strong connection to the ground and a source of solidity for manipulation. Let's go a little deeper into how you can be aware of your body.

Taking your center and limbs into account, you can mentally divide the body into four quarters, with a line vertically up the center and horizontally across the center of mass. As we're symmetrical beings, this more or less divides the body into four equally weighted segments, and uses the spine as a focal point for where muscles attach. In fact, there are very few muscles that cross over the centerline of the body. You could make an argument that the rectus abdominis (abs) covers the entire front of the body, but it is clearly segmented down the middle. Even most muscles of the head are delineated on the left and right side.

In the horizontal direction, cutting across the center of mass, the rectus abdominis again crosses this boundary (remember how important this muscle is?) as does the latissimus dorsi (the muscle around your lower back), and the interior muscles around the spine like the longissimus, iliocostalis, multifidus, and a few others. Notably, the only muscle to connect the legs to the spine is the psoas muscle (covered in the anatomy section), so there is a pretty good separation in the upper and lower parts of the body as well.

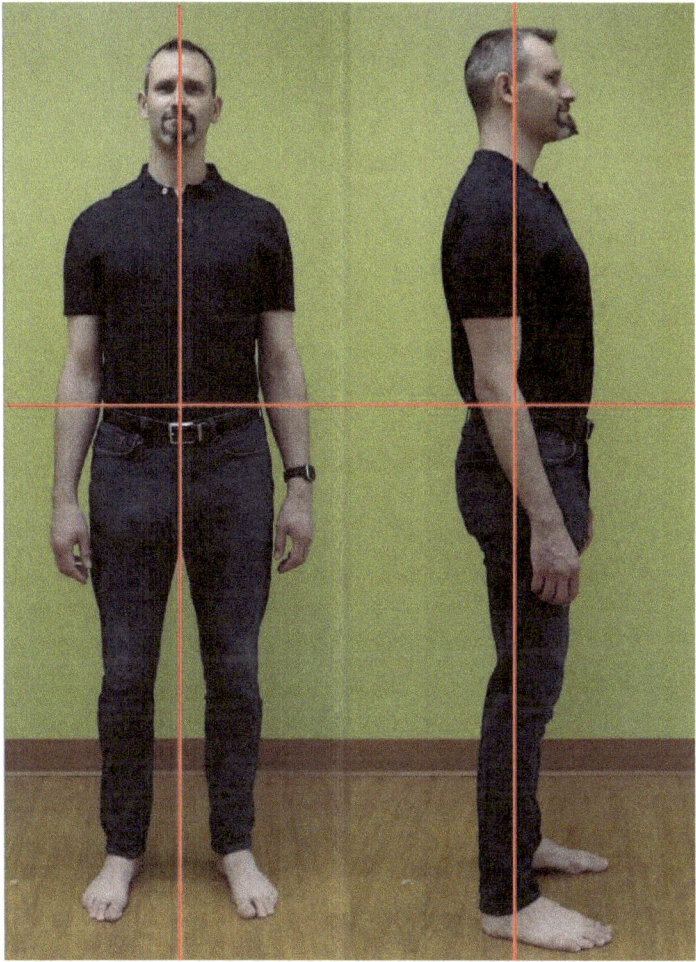

Figure 96: The human body can be divided into quarters, which can operate independently.

What does this mean, and why am I devoting the final section of this book to it? Because we typically think of our bodies as monolithic. It moves all together or not at all, but this isn't really the case. Here's a last exercise for you to play with, which involves using your core muscles, the interior muscles around the spine, the larger back muscles, the big muscles around the glutes and pelvis, and more.

Try to move one quarter of your body without moving the rest.

It doesn't have to be a big or complex movement. Try curling one arm, shoulder, collarbone, and pectoral inward, while leaving the rest of your body motionless. Maybe go backward instead. This might be harder with legs if you're standing up, but you can stand on one leg and manipulate the other in the air without moving your arms or your support leg. Your pelvic and shoulder joints are independently mobile, so you can twist one leg inward while the other is straight, and the same for the shoulder joints. Take all those exercises with the spine and try to only move the muscles on one side of the spine, not both.

You won't get this immediately, and that's okay. But once you do, you can manufacture an incredible stability in the rest of your body while only moving one quarter of it. This is a great way to apply extra muscle to a task. For example, find a doorway where you can grasp it in one hand. Like the exercises above concerning moving your muscles against each other, push and pull on the doorway (using good barrel!) and you can move your body forward and backward easily. Now, try to isolate the one quarter of your body gripping the doorframe. Keep the rest of your body from moving, but still pull and push on the door! What you're doing is moving the motion internal to your body, building power from your (immobile) core. Imagine applying this same power to hammering a nail or lifting a heavy box of goods on a shelf. Keep your core in mind, whatever you're doing. The more you know how to operate your body, the more you will have absolute control over it. This is the basis of complex activities like martial arts, bellydancing, gymnastics, professional sports, and many others.

> Being able to control only a single muscle is an extraordinary feat! Singling out a few muscles in a group you usually move all at once is even harder.

As a final note, don't just take my examples as the only thing you can do with these tips and tricks. Play around with them. Do them so much they are encoded in your muscle memory. Then, when you do an unfamiliar action, one of these might come out, whether it's using a barrel, or walking sideways, or lifting a heavy object, or stopping a fall.

In fact, that might be the main takeaway from this book. Even if you didn't do the exercises (but you did do them all, didn't you?), you should still have a better understanding of how your body works. Hopefully some of these ideas have sunk in, and one or two of them might come out and surprise you one of these days.

Wrap-up

Well, that was a lot! Congratulations on learning how to operate your body.

If you have gone through the exercises, I hope you've learned a lot about the way your body works. Simply standing up straight is a big step to easing back, knee, and other joint pain. Learning how to approach and lift objects will save you a lot in shoulder and neck pain. While I go on about moving efficiently, moving *correctly* is just as important. I see a lot of people in pain while they move around. I see a lot of others who don't necessarily have joint pain, but I can tell their body will degrade faster because they are not using it properly. You've taken a big step in coming this far.

If you like the examples in this book, I've put together a series of videos along with the other teachers at my martial arts school. We take these concepts, and some others I haven't covered, in three-to-five-minute clips. If you've enjoyed this book, I think you'll enjoy them too. You can find them here: https://www.youtube.com/@howtooperateyourbody6460

These tips and tricks can help you, but only if you take the time to learn what I've shown here. Just imagine learning how to operate your feet, legs, arms, hands, and head! If you do that, there is a whole other series of actions that you can do with your entire body, rather than just part of it.

Remember, practice makes perfect. That's a trite saying, but it became a cliché because it's true. I touched on muscle memory during this book, and it's a big part of how you live your daily life. You don't think about how every little muscle moves until you start learning a new skill. Then you suddenly become aware of whatever body part you're using to do that new skill.

I want you to get to a place where you're constantly questioning how your body moves and never falling into a routine. Even if you've committed good posture to muscle memory, and you think you always stand up straight, take a second or two to check now and then. You may find your body has tricked you and decided to go back to some old habit. This can be frustrating and feels like you're taking a step backward rather than forward. The fact that you noticed it means you're learning! So don't despair. Because there isn't a convenient manual, it takes a lifetime to truly learn how to operate your body. Your success is measured by every single step you take, forward, back, or sideways. Your success is measured by *doing* it, rather than by ignoring your body, and hoping it stops bothering you. Keep at it.

One more option! I teach all this in my martial arts class. If you live near Raleigh, NC, and are interested in joining my school, I welcome anyone who is interested in changing their life for the better. You can find more information here: https://sites.google.com/site/raleighwado/

I also run an online workshop where I will personally teach you how to operate your body. Just go to my Patreon page at https://www.patreon.com/wctracy Think of it like reading this book, but you can ask me questions while you're doing it, and I can tell you all the things I forgot or didn't have time to put in here.

I hope you liked this book. If you learned even one new thing, I'll count that as a success. I love teaching, because every so often I see that look on a student's face that tells me they've *gotten* it. If you have that same epiphany, please let me know. You can email me at wctracy@williamctracy.com. In addition, if you thought you gained something from this book, please leave a review at the bookseller where you purchased it. You'll be helping other people make the same decision you did and take the first step in learning How to Operate Your Body.

ACKNOWLEDGEMENTS

This book was meant to be three books. I released *How to Operate Your Body: The Legs* in 2024, and meant to write another book on The Arms, then The Core. However in writing about the arms, I found there was so much material that depended on knowing how to use your legs, I would have ended up repeating half the book. The core depends on both arms and legs, so I decided to put all three of these books together in one volume. I hope you get something useful out of it!

The concept for this came from being a writer, an engineer, and a martial artist. Sometimes, I have to be told not to stare at people when they let me out of the house. I'm either staring because the person will make a great character in a book, or because I'm trying to understand how they're interacting with the world and using/misusing some piece of technology, or because some part of the way they walk or move has caught my attention. You'd be surprised how often it's the last one. Eventually, I decided to write a book about it.

Thanks first go to my co-teachers, Josiah and Courtney Brooks, for helping with concepting this book and developing the online videos for How to Operate Your Body (or as we fondly call it, HTOYB). As we've taught martial arts, we've found it matters less the system you start with, and more how the human body moves. We've all got the same basic body concept, and understanding how joints and muscles move means understanding the possibilities that we don't always take advantage of. I've had some fantastic martial arts instructors, mentioned in the forward, and I continue to have new eureka moments with body mechanics the more I practice.

I want to thank all my fellow martial artists, both peers and students. I've learned many times more while teaching than practicing on my own. Also thank you Scott, Greg, and TJ for some early examples of how not to walk, and my father for how not to lift things. ;-)

Thanks as always to my beta readers, who tell me when I'm not making any sense, and lastly, but never least, to my copy editor (and wife) Heather for fixing all my writing mistakes.

ABOUT THE AUTHOR

William C. Tracy writes and publishes queer science fiction and fantasy through his indie press Space Wizard Science Fantasy (spacewizardsciencefantasy.com).

His largest work is the Dissolutionverse: a space opera with music-based magic, including ten books and an RPG. He also has a standalone epic fantasy with seasonal fruit-based magic, this nonfiction book about body mechanics and correct posture, and a hard sci-fi trilogy with generational colony ships and a planet covered by a sentient fungal entity. He's currently working on a progression fantasy series about martial arts and moving islands.

William is an NC native and a lifelong fan of science fiction and fantasy. He has a master's degree in mechanical engineering, and has both designed and operated heavy construction machinery. He has also trained in Wado-Ryu karate since 2003 and runs his own dojo in Raleigh, NC. He is an avid video and board gamer, a beekeeper, a reader, and of course, a writer.

You can get a free Dissolutionverse novelette by signing up for William's mailing list at spacewizardsciencefantasy.com

Follow him on Bluesky at wctracy.bsky.social, Threads at threads.net/@tracywc, and Twitter at @wctracy for writing updates, cat and bee pictures, and thoughts on martial arts.

Please take a moment to review this book at your favorite retailer's website, Goodreads, or simply tell your friends!